Forget the Vet

Homeopathic Remedies for Cats & Dogs Including Recipes

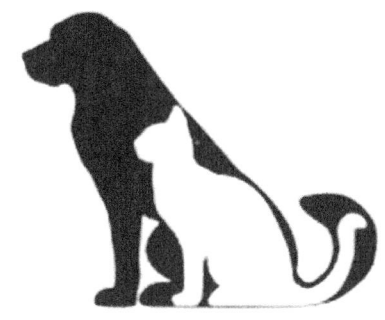

Pennie Mae Cartawick

Important Legal Disclaimer:

The information presented in this book reflects the author's opinions and is by no way intended as medical advice or as a substitute for medical counseling. This information should be used in conjunction with the guidance and care of your veterinarian. Consult your vet before starting your pet on any exercise and nutrition program.

The author has made every effort to supply accurate information in the creation of this book. The author offers no warranty and accepts no responsibility for any loss, allergic reactions, or damages of any kind that may be incurred by an animal as a result of actions arising from the use of the contents in this book. If you choose not to obtain the consent of your vet and/or work with your veterinarian throughout the duration of your time using the recommendations in this book, you are agreeing to accept full responsibility for your actions.

All rights reserved, no part of this book may be used, reproduced, or transmitted in any form or by any means without the expressed written permission of the author.

First edition. Copyright 2015

Pennie Mae Cartawick

Table of Contents

Introduction	1
Pet Diabetes	4
Causes of cat and dog diabetes:	4
Symptoms of a diabetic cat or dog:	5
Herbal Remedies.	6
Diabetic recipes.	11
Grocery list for Diabetic Pets.	18
Homemade Raw Food for Cats with Kidney Problems.	21
The Recipe.	22
Herbal Solutions.	25
Homeopathic Remedies for Cats with Constipation.	27
Cats and Allergies.	30
Natural Cure/Remedy:	31
Homemade Cat Recipes.	35
Dental Health.	43
Bladder Problems.	44
Herbal Remedies.	46
Cats with Colds and Flu Symptoms.	47
Cats, Head to Paw.	50
Flea and tick repellent.	55
Weight Loss	58
Cat Body Condition Chart.	58
Grocery Shopping List for Cats	62
Pets and Tapeworms.	66
Natural remedies using Homeopathy	66

Recipes	68
Home Treatments for Dental Health.	70
Homemade Healthy Dental Treats:	72
The Holistic Approach to Dog Ailments.	75
Overall Nutrition:	82
Homemade Dog Food & Treats	83
Time to cut out the junk.	88
Is your dog over weight?	88
Dog Condition Weight Chart	90
Easy ways to have an effective weight loss program for your Dog.	91
Healthy recipes for your Dog.	93
Grocery Shopping List for Dogs.	98
Dogs with Asthma: What you need to know	101
Herbal Remedies.	102
Index	114
Author	118
Books	119

Introduction

Forget the Vet' focuses on the many health benefits of practicing natural remedies. Cooking easy homemade holistic recipes, and treating your pet to a homeopathic agenda, may prevent many trips to your vet's office.

A note from the author: I wasn't blessed with children, so animals became the biggest part of my life. Many years ago, my cat named 'Odi' was diagnosed with allergies, asthma, and a heart murmur. Finding the right treatments for him became a priority. I very nearly went to the vet so he could be treated with a steroid injection to relieve his breathing issues, that is, until I found out that such an injection can cause diabetes. This was the start of finding other alternative methods to traditional medicine. This book was made possible through a lot of dedicated research into finding treatments for my much loved companion 'Odi'. After all, the health and vitality of our pets is essential as they are a big part of our lives.

A combination that counts: When we look holistically at all the natural cures for ailments in our pets, we ask ourselves, should we go all natural or use supplements that contain processed ingredients? There is no hard or fast rule to this. It is obvious that most products that come from natural sources have higher levels for benefiting our pets than others. The combination of processed substances and natural sources only arise due to the shortage of natural materials in certain locations. It is important to always use products that are as natural as possible. This saves the stress of getting your pets hooked on medications that may do them more harm than good. For instance, steroid injections used to treat Asthma hold ingredients that may cause Diabetes. The way you treat your pets and groom them, goes a long way in determining their overall health.

A Smart move to make.

This book lists a few of the natural cures for common ailments in pets. Some of the ingredients listed here are preventive, while others are curative. What is essential, is to help your pets live longer, and for them to lead fuller healthier lives.

ODI

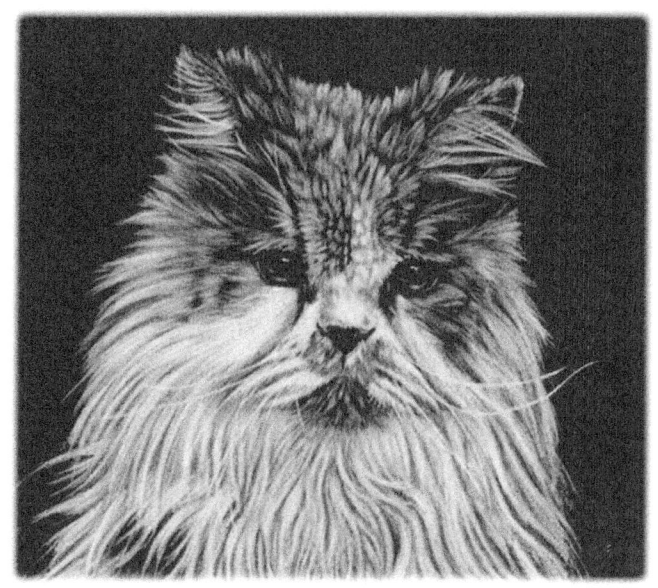

Pet Diabetes

Pets, just like ourselves, are at a significant risk of developing diabetes. Research shows that approximately one in every 400 cats and one in 500 dogs are very likely to suffer from Diabetes. Diabetes can lead to many complications; among them, liver and kidney disease, heart disease, coma and even death. Cats and dogs are the most common of pets in our homes so pet owners should learn about various issues concerning diabetes.

Causes of cat and dog diabetes:

What brings forth cases of diabetes in pets is very similar to that of ourselves. The pancreas organ in the body produces a hormone called insulin. Insulin ensures the blood sugar in the body is balanced. Sometimes the pancreas is not able to produce enough insulin and this affects the balancing of the blood sugar as well as the glucose levels within the body. Dogs are at high risk of getting Diabetes type 1, which is mainly caused by the pancreas not being able to secrete enough insulin. To help treat dogs from type 1 of diabetes, insulin therapy is recommended. Cats are at a higher risk of getting type 2 diabetes which is caused by the lack of proper response to insulin.

Research shows that the major cause of diabetes in cats and dogs is the high sugar content in commercial processed foods. Some factors such as obesity, an unhealthy diet, and stress can all contribute to the high likelihood of pets getting diabetes. It can also be genetic, hence hereditary. Pet owners in most cases do not know what symptoms to look for in diabetes.

Symptoms of a diabetic cat or dog:

1. Weight loss.

Any pet that sheds a lot of weight, especially in a short amount of time becomes a point of concern and it may signify a medical problem. Lack of appetite is a major cause of weight loss in diabetic animals. In most cases, cats are unable to utilize the calories they eat and because of this, they begin to break down their body fats to gain energy loss. As the fat breaks down, the cat sheds a lot of weight.

2. Frequent urination.

Polyuria is the term used to describe the abnormal frequency of urinating in cats and dogs. Polyuria and polydipsia go hand in hand. It is very important to have the veterinary check your pet to rule out any doubt on diabetes.

3. Excessive thirst.

Excessive drinking of water is a common sign of diabetes. This condition is referred to as polydipsia.

4. Change in appetite.

Some diabetic pets tend to have a poor appetite while others have an increased appetite. The bottom line is, if your pet eats more or less of the normal amounts, it is important to seek medical advice.

5. Changed walking style.

Some diabetic cats change the way they walk with their paws landing on the ground different than usual. An abnormality of their nervous systems causes this.

6. Depression.

Just like us, cats and dogs also suffer from depression. This condition is referred to as Ketoacidosis. This is caused by fats and proteins in the liver breaking down as a response to the lack of insulin. Weakness and fatigue may characterize depression. Signs include weakness, especially in the back legs of most cats. Dogs tend to be less active and sleep more than usual.

7. Vomiting.

If your pet has persistent vomiting, it goes without saying that there may be an underlying medical problem that may include diabetes.

8. Thinning Fur.

Some cats and dogs tend to have dull, thinning and shedding of fur. This may be a sign of a medical problem that includes diabetes.

9. Cataracts.

This refers to cloudy eyes, especially in dogs. These cloudy eyes may be a sign of early diabetes in dogs and it should be monitored closely as it could lead to blindness.

Some of these symptoms are also present in other types of illnesses. A blood sugar test is necessary to diagnose the right ailment or disease.

Herbal Remedies.

Diabetes in cats and dogs if not treated early enough, can lead to fatality. Simple natural remedies can help prevent or help treat diabetic pets. Healthy nutrition is important to eliminate the chances of having a diabetic cat or dog. An overweight pet is unhealthy and may lead to early stages of Diabetes. A strict diet as well as a lot of exercise needs to become a regular routine. Research shows that a diet that is low in carbohydrate and rich in protein is suitable.

Herbal treatments:

Most veterinarians recommend natural remedies for animals suffering from diabetes.

a) **Galego Officinalis** - This natural ingredient improves the part of the pancreas that produces insulin.

b) **Chromium** - This aids in balancing cholesterol within the body. Chromium also ensures that the insulin in the body is effective.

c) **Bilberry** - This ingredient is known to minimize glucose levels in pets suffering from type 2 diabetes. Research also indicates that bilberry helps improve vision as well as aiding wounds to heal quickly.

Homeopathic cures.

Homeopathy simply refers to treatment of a disease by using natural substances (plant extracts) that aids and treat symptoms in your pet.

Below are some easy homeopathic remedies.

PLANTAGO OVATA.

Otherwise known as 'blond plantain' and 'Desert Indian wheat'. This plant has quite a bit of mucilage, even more so than flax seed. Mucilage is a thick, gooey substance that is actually soluble fiber in a viscous form. Fiber rich foods slow the absorption of carbohydrates and this helps prevent sudden spikes in blood sugar levels. Mucilage is highly beneficial for diabetic cats as its texture is easy for them to absorb when compared with other sources of fiber.

CRANBERRY AND BLUEBERRY EXTRACT.

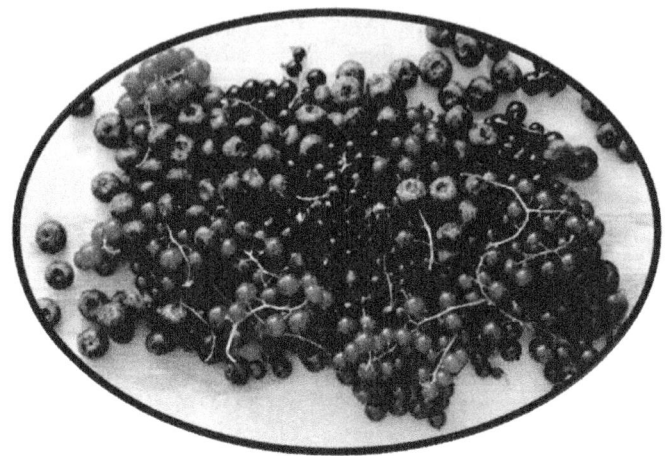

Both of these fruit extracts are used in the treatment of diabetes in cats as they both contain powerful anti-oxidants while boosting the immune system. As diabetic cats are overly susceptible to pests and infections, they need all the immunological support they can get.

CHROMIUM PICOLINATE.

This is an easily absorbed form of Chromium, a chemical element that is present in organs and acts as a nutrient that is essential for the proper metabolism of sugars and fats. Correct pancreatic functioning depends on the proper metabolism of sugar and fat. Chromium Pico Linate helps with the efficiency of insulin within the body.

NOPAL CACTUS.

This wild plant comes from colder desert regions. It is an extremely nutritious plant that is appropriate for animal consumption. In fact, the pet food brand IAMS sells a dehydrated Nopal Cactus blend. Regarding diabetes, it has been shown that Nopal Cactus increases levels of natural insulin within the body, and thus stabilizes blood sugar levels. It also reduces concentrations of glucose, cholesterol, and triglycerides in the blood.

OMEGA 3.

Omega 3 fatty acid aids in dryness of the skin, and its anti-inflammatory properties help with arthritic pain that is common in diabetic cats. Natural sources of Omega 3 include fish such as salmon, sardines, anchovies, and herring.

FLAX OIL.

This is also a good source although cats are not able to handle excessive amounts. Although many major pet food brands claim that they add Omega 3 to their dry and wet cat food, the truth is that the high temperature cooking that is a necessary part of the packaging process actually degrades the Omega 3 oils that are added to the food. Thus, it is much better to feed your cat a natural source of Omega 3 by capsule form. Omega 3 can be found at any health food store. Just break the capsule and add it to your pet's food.

FENUGREEK SEEDS.

These small, yellow seeds are cultivated mainly in India. This plant has many medicinal properties that are of particular significance to diabetic cats: it helps to control cholesterol, fights against obesity, and for older female cats, it can even alleviate the symptoms of menopause. It also contains flavonoid routine, which improves the overall health of your cat, and combats the effects of ocular degeneration that are typically associated with diabetes. Nonetheless, when giving this plant to your cat, it is extremely important not to overuse it as this may cause serious side effects.

TURMERIC ROOT.

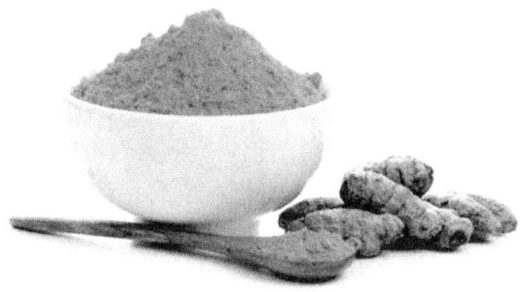

This root belongs to the ginger family. Turmeric Root supplements are particularly recommended for diabetic pets who are insulin resistant. It is an extremely effective as an anti-inflammatory, and it helps to reduce body weight in over weight animals. It is a natural analgesic that alieves all ailments of aches and pains that our fury friends are susceptible too as they age. It is also an antiseptic and antibiotic treatment, and it helps with liver problems, pancreatic cancer, and rheumatism. Basically, I could go on and on as to the health benefits of Turmeric Root; its many heath promoting properties have been known to date back to ancient times.

GYMNEMA SYLVESTRE.

This plant is often referred to as a 'sugar destroyer' and in centuries past, it was one of the herbal remedies that was most sought after in order to treat diabetes. Its properties also help stabilize hyperactivity, rheumatism, hemorrhoids, and many other conditions related to improper sugar metabolism. Gymnema Sylestre protects the liver, controls cholesterol, indigestion, and aids gastric problems. This plant extract produces insulin which aids to increase pancreatic beta cells.

BEER YEAST.

Since diabetes and vitamin deficiency often go hand in hand, it's important to make sure that a diabetic animal is still getting all the vitamins and minerals he/she needs to stay healthy and active. Beer yeast is an excellent choice. This nutritional supplement is chock full of vitamins and minerals. It contains a whole host of B vitamins, folic acid, chromium, iron, zinc, and lots of healthy proteins. It aids with the metabolism of fats and carbohydrates, and as such, helps our furry friends keep their energy levels high for longer periods of time. Many pets benefit from beer yeast, but be aware that there are some pets that are allergic to beer yeast. If you notice that they seem to be scratching themselves more than usual after consuming beer yeast, he/she may suffer with an allergic. The recommended quantity is one teaspoon spoonful per day.

Diabetic recipes.

Diabetic pets need a strict diet. Below are a few recipes that are appropriate ones for diabetes. Pet owners should note that these recipes may not be suitable for certain dogs and cats. A consultation with a veterinarian may be necessary before indulging in any of the recipes below. Alterations of these recipes can be made to the suitability of the pet.

Recipe one:

Ingredients

- 6 lb. lean meat, either beef or chicken
- 5 cups raw pearl barley
- 5 cups raw brown rice
- 5 cups vegetables - you can use minced celery, spinach, green beans.
- 24 cups of water - a cup of brown rice takes two cups of water while a cup of barley takes three cups of water.

Method

Place all the above ingredients in to a sizeable pot. Let them boil over a medium heat. Remove from heat when all the water is absorbed. This method produces around 2 gallons of food.

Recipe two:

Ingredients

- 4 cups raw brown rice
- 3 cups carrots (chopped)
- 2 cups celery (chopped)
- 1 bunch of broccoli
- 1 bunch of fresh spinach
- 110 oz. of meat (beef or chicken)
- 3 cloves of garlic (crushed)
- 3 cups raw rye

Method

Cook the meat and garlic in water for about 20 minutes. Remove the beef from the broth and add the rye. Cover and boil the rye for about 40 minutes. Add the rice and simmer for approximately 15 minutes. In a large pot, mix the raw vegetables in with the meat. Then add the hot rye and rice over the vegetables and mix well. The hot rice and rye steams the vegetables ensuring the retention of nutrients from cooking.

This recipe takes 25% vegetables, 25% protein (lean beef, chicken or fish) and 50% carbohydrates.

Recipe three:

Ingredients

- 1 cup of oatmeal
- 1 cup of natural wheat bran
- 1/2 cup of wheat germ
- 1 cup of peanut (chopped in a blender)
- 1 egg
- 1 cup of water

Method

Preheat the oven to 350 degrees. Mix all the ingredients in a large pot. Roll the mixture into approximately twelve balls, and place them on an ungreased sheet then bake for approximately 15 minutes. When ready, allow them to cool. Store in the freezer.

Peanuts help to control the oxygen flow in the cells. They contain iron, folic acid, calcium, potassium, magnesium among other nutrients. Wheat germ contains vitamin E, calcium, magnesium, copper and phosphorous.

Recipe four:

Ingredients

- Cooked meat, either chicken or beef (skinless)
- Whole wheat bread
- Water

Method

Mash all the ingredients together and then roll them up into pepperoni size. Freeze the rolls in sandwich bags. Always serve frozen to your pet.

Recipe five:

Ingredients

- 2 large whole chicken breasts (skinless)
- 1 bunch of Broccoli
- 2 cups raw brown rice

Method

Boil the chicken in enough water and save the broth. When the chicken is ready, remove from heat and cut into small pieces. Cook the rice in 5 cups of broth for approximately 25 minutes. Steam the broccoli separately then combine the chicken, rice, and broccoli and mix well. Water can be added if it seems a little too dry.

Recipe six:

Ingredients

- 1/4 kg lean beef
- 1/2 cup un-creamed, low-fat cheese (your choice of cheese)
- 3 cups fresh and chopped green beans (stems should be removed)
- 7 grams bone meal (this may be bought from any health food store)

Method

Cook beef in a sizeable pan. Stir lightly until brown. Add the remaining ingredients and mix them together. When ready, serve. Place the remainder in the refrigerator using an airtight container.

Recipe seven:

Ingredients

- 1 cup of uncooked white rice
- 1/2 cup minced or ground raw chicken
- 1/2 tablespoonful corn oil
- 1/2 cup green beans or sliced carrots (either fresh or frozen)
- 1/4 teaspoonful salt
- 5 grams of bone meal (Can be purchased from any health store)

Method

Mix rice, salt, and corn oil with twice the volume of boiling water. Cook for about 15 minutes. Add the remaining ingredients and mix well. Simmer for 10 minutes.

This recipe makes enough food for two days.

Recipe eight:

Ingredients

- 1 cup cooked pasta
- 1 cup minced raw chicken
- 1 cup teaspoon corn oil
- 1 cup green beans
- ¼ teaspoon salt
- 3.75 grams Di-calcium phosphate

Method

Sauté the chicken in the oil. Steam the vegetables. Mix the chicken, vegetables and pasta with the remaining ingredients. Let it cool and then refrigerate in an airtight container.

This recipe makes enough food for two days.

Tips.

Pet owners should always check the sugar labels and buy the leanest meats possible. Semi-moist foods should be avoided because of their high possible sugar content.

Tips to remember while administering insulin.

1. Insulin should always be stored in the refrigerator.

2. Insulin should be mixed using a gentle rolling method before being used and should never be shaken.

3. Expired insulin should never be used.

4. Shave the fur of the pet's area previous to injecting them.

Contributors to high risk of diabetes.

Any pet can get diabetes. Some animals are at a higher risk of getting diabetes than others. These factors include but are not limited to:

Age. Older pets are more likely to get diabetes as opposed to younger ones.

Certain breeds. Siamese cats, are at a higher risk of being diabetic than other breeds.

Overweight pets are also more at risk from developing Diabetes.

Lack of exercise.

An unhealthy diet in pets that contains too much sugar.

The bottom line.

It is evident that pet's diabetes is treatable when a regimen is started early. It is, however, good to note that prevention is better than a cure. Pet owners should learn to prevent chances of cats and dogs getting diabetes and they should be monitored by the provision of a healthy diet and by administering regular exercise. Exercise serves its own purpose through eliminating excess sugars within the body. Above all, sugar is the main food for diabetes. Sugar should be eliminated in all pet's meals. A sugarless diet is all that pets require to have a diabetic free life.

Grocery list for Diabetic Pets.

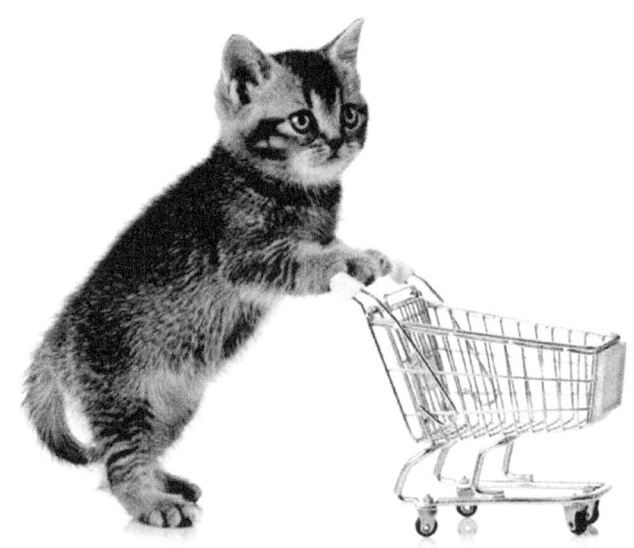

Meat.

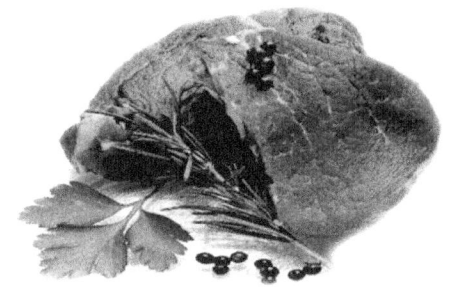

Chicken/Beef

Produce.

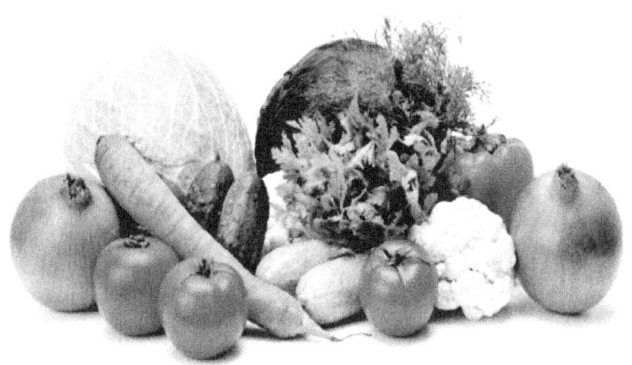

Carrots
Spinach
Celery
Broccoli
Green beans

Poultry.

Eggs
Cheese (low fat)

Grains/Nuts/Other.

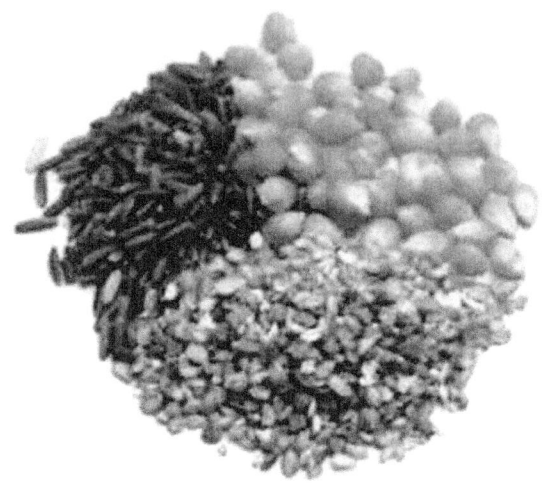

Raw Rye
Wheat/White bread
Peanuts
Oatmeal
Wheat Bran
Wheat Germ
Barley
Pasta
Salt
Di- Calcium Phosphate
Bone Meal
Corn oil
Garlic

Homemade Raw Food for Cats with Kidney Problems.

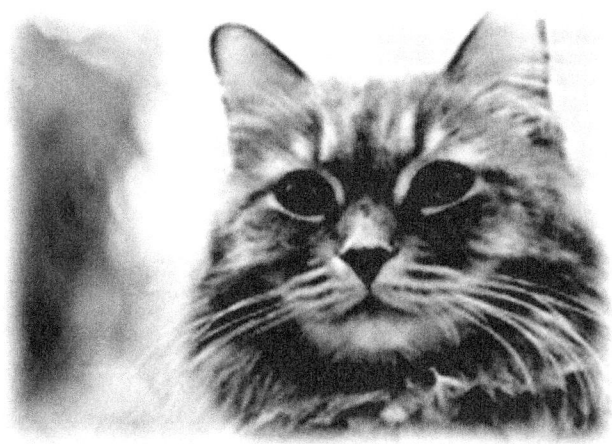

Contrary to what you may have heard, cats with kidney problems do need protein. However, they need high quality protein that has the right ratio of amino acids and is low in phosphorus and sodium. Organic chicken, rabbit, hare, and possum are the best sources of protein for cats with chronic kidney problems.

Store bought dried cat food has very high levels of phosphorous and sodium, but healthy cats can deal with this by concentrating these compounds in their urine tract and eliminating it. Cats with kidney problems are extremely common, especially with the Persian breed.

Below is a simple homemade recipe that is low in phosphorus and sodium which is suitable for cats with kidney problems. You will have enough food to last approximately two weeks. All you need is a pot, a high powered blender, and some items that you can buy at a specialty butcher and/or the supermarket. Additionally, I have added a list of extra items that you can add to this basic recipe for additional nutritional and therapeutic benefits.

The Recipe.

Boil water in a pot and drop in two skinless legs and thighs from a whole chicken. Once they begin to change color, remove them. This should take about a minute. You don't want to cook the meat as this will remove valuable nutrients; the only reason that you are boiling the meat is to kill any bacteria. You want to use legs and thighs because these parts of the chicken or rabbit have the right amount of fat and contain a substance called taurine. Taurine helps regulate the right levels of bile which is essential for cats that have malfunctioning kidneys. In fact, felines absolutely need taurine in their diet, and when they don't get enough, this can lead to retinal degeneration and irreversible blindness.

Once you've taken out the legs and thighs, keep the water boiling, and add the offal, specifically the liver, heart, and gizzards. Use a ladle, as you only want to dip these organs into the boiling water for five seconds at the most. Again, the boiling water is only there to kill the bacteria. If you let these organs cook longer, they will harden and take on a flavor that is unappetizing to most cats. Cats are notoriously picky eaters and even more so when they are sick. Next, you want to add a piece of fish for additional omega 3, preferably salmon, fresh tuna, or bream. However, as these types of fish can be expensive, you may use sardines or any other river fish that hasn't been factory farmed. Factory farmed produce contains considerably less nutrients than organic. Again, in order to avoid losing nutrients, you want to boil the fish very quickly, until it just barely starts to change color. Another way to kill bacteria is to oven bake the meat or fish at 180 degrees for a few minutes. Some people choose to avoid the use of heat altogether, and use unsweetened citrus, natural lemon, or grapefruit juice to disinfect the meat.

Once everything has been cooked (albeit barely cooked) it's time to throw everything in the blender. How much blending you do will depend entirely on the particular taste of your cat. Ideally, it would be better to have a consistency that contains larger chunks. This way, the cat will chew it which helps clean their teeth. Nonetheless, some cats won't go near their food unless it's nice and mushy.

As you're blending the meat, you can add a very small amount of fresh fruit or vegetables. For example, choose one of the following options:

An eighth of an apple or a pear

- 2 cranberries
- 2 raspberries
- A fifth of a tomato
- Half a spinach leaf.

Again, you only want to choose one of these options!

You may grind up the bones, but make sure that you have the right kind of bender to do this. Bones contain lots of healthy calcium, but sharp bone fragments especially from Chicken, can be extremely dangerous, and can cause life threatening intestinal ruptures.

Once everything has been blended, divide into daily portions inside plastic bags and freeze it. Regular cats can eat between 70 and 100 grams on a daily basis.

Ideally, the finished blended cat food should contain 70 percent thigh and leg, 20 percent fish, with only very small amounts of whatever fruit or vegetable you decide to use. Change up the fruit/vegetable you use from time to time, and do the same with the meat and fish. Our pets enjoy variety as much as we do.

Additional items.

In order to add variety to your cat's meal and also provide valuable nutrition that helps with kidney problems, related urinary tract issues, and other health issues, you can add the following items, supplements, and herbs.

Protein.

We have already mentioned organic chicken, organic rabbit, and wild caught fish (canned tuna is not a good option for cats with renal problems). Cats with a more advanced kidney degeneration should avoid red meat as it will be hard to metabolize. Other safe sources of protein include quail, and soft-cooked eggs. Cats are carnivores, and all of their meals should be protein based, never carbohydrate based.

Fruits and Vegetables.

Cats in the wild do not naturally eat fruits or vegetables, however they do benefit from vegetable matter and seeds that are found in the stomachs of their prey. As a result, domesticated cats should also be fed small quantities of certain fruits and vegetables. These include; apples, pears, carrots, spinach, broccoli, alfalfa, seaweed, kelp, raspberries, blueberries, and cranberries. Avoid dehydrated berries as these contain unhealthy amounts of sugar. Also, grapes and raisins must be avoided and although it is not entirely understood as to why, grapes and raisins can actually cause acute kidney failure in cats that are otherwise perfectly healthy. Onion is also toxic for cats.

Fats.

All pets need healthy fats. Good sources of nutritious fat that you can add to your homemade cat food include; fish oil, canola oil, and sunflower seed oil.

Herbal Solutions.

Rosemary. This is another herb that is great for cats. Most love the taste of Rosemary, so if you find that your sick cat is not eating enough, then adding some rosemary to its food will make it more palatable. It also stimulates the circulatory system.

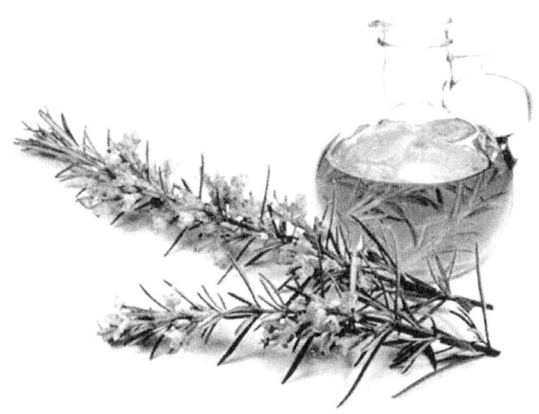

Flax Seed (Omega 3) Cats with kidney problems already have compromised immune systems, and flax seed helps control reactions to flea bites. It also helps to maintain healthy fur.

Soy Lecithin Helps emulsify cholesterol, and helps with the digestion and absorption of fats.

Linoleic Acid (Omega 6) Cats with defective kidneys have problems regulating moisture and this supplement helps keep their skin and fur lubricated and moist.

Sage. Impaired neurological functions are symptoms of elevated levels of phosphorus that are common with cats with kidney problems. This can be combated with sage as this herb aids cats with cognitive functions.

Thyme. This is a powerful natural antibiotic that also fights parasites.

Amaranth. Amaranth is loaded with vitamins, it also helps to calm the stomach, and reduces the inflammation of soft tissues. However, as it is a grain, and cats are not suited to eating lots of carbohydrates, it should only be given in moderation.

Beer Yeast. Not only does this contain 16 amino acids and plenty of vitamins and minerals, it also helps cats eliminate toxins. This is important for cats with damaged kidneys as their livers have to work overtime.

Chicory Root. If you have a cat that has especially foul smelling feces, adding chicory root can help alleviate this problem.

Using natural plant extracts really does improve the quality of your beloved pet's life. You will notice an improvement in your cat's well-being within weeks after you change their diet and add homeopathic remedies to their meal plan. Should your cat continue to have symptoms of kidney failure, consult with your veterinarian.

Homeopathic Remedies for Cats with Constipation.

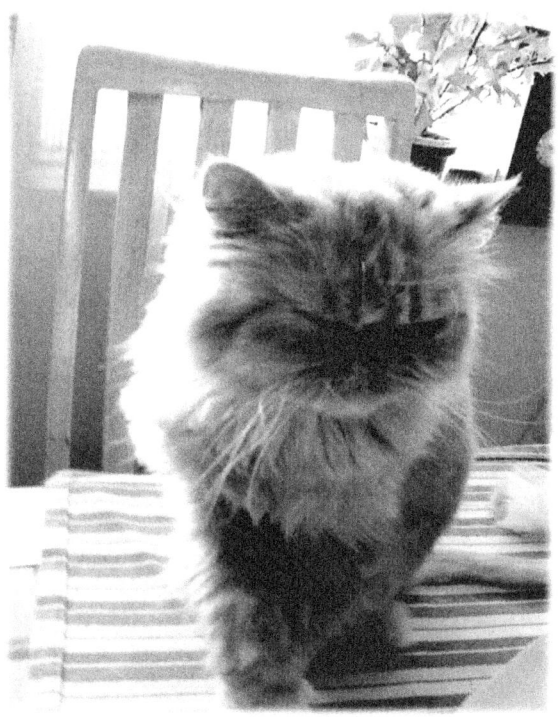

Pumpkin.

When a cat is constipated and needs a specialized diet to get their bowels moving again, one of the hardest aspects you face, is that they can be extremely finicky when it comes to what they eat. Thankfully, a natural laxative that most cats tend to like, is the taste of raw organic pumpkin. Since pumpkin already has a soft texture, it requires basically no preparation; simply stir a spoonful into your cat's food once daily.

Farmer's Market Organic pumpkin is one of the best brands, as it is USDA approved, and contains no harmful preservatives. The actual can it comes in is free of the dangerous toxin called Bisphenol A. This chemical is often found in cans including many supermarket cat foods. Whatever you do, make sure not to give your cat pumpkin pie filling, as this contains a lot of sugar and other ingredients that can make your already constipated cat, seriously ill.

Fiber.

When we are constipated, we remedy the situation by adding fiber to our diet. Cats are no different. However, there are several kinds of fiber, and certain types can actually aggravate a cat's constipation and pain.

When it comes to your cat, there are three types of fiber that can alleviate constipation; Insoluble fibers such as wheat bran and oat fiber, soluble fibers such as guar gum and oat bran, and mixed fibers such as pea fiber and beet pulp.

Whichever source of fiber you choose, start off small using one teaspoon mixed with their food twice daily; you don't want all of the compacted feces within their body to start moving too quickly all at once, as this can not only be painful, but can cause cuts, tears, and even infection. Make sure to give the fiber some time to work which may be as long as three days.

Lubricants for your cat.

If pumpkin and fiber don't seem to do the trick, then it may be time to consider a natural stool softener.

Evenly distribute drops of olive oil - a tablespoon's worth will do. Douse it all over your cat's wet cat food (don't exacerbate a constipation problem by feeding your cat kibble). Vegetable oil or oil based canned tuna may also work. Although this is not the best thing to give your cat, canned tuna is a tasty, once-in-a-while treat that your cat will really enjoy. Make sure that their food is not drenched in oil though!

Dairy.

Contrary to the popular story book image of a content kitty lapping up a saucer full of milk, the truth of the matter is, cats are lactose intolerant. Cats, especially older cats, lack an enzyme called lactase in their digestive tract. This is the enzyme that is needed to break down the lactose contained in milk and all dairy products such as cheese, yogurt and eggs. Giving pets dairy products will result in diarrhea.

Nonetheless, when your cat's intestines are backed up, a dose of dairy may just be exactly what it needs. One eighth of a cup of whole milk twice a day for a couple of days will be sufficient to counteract this ailment. Once your cat's bowel movements are back to normal, slowly ween him/her off the dairy.

Cats and Allergies.

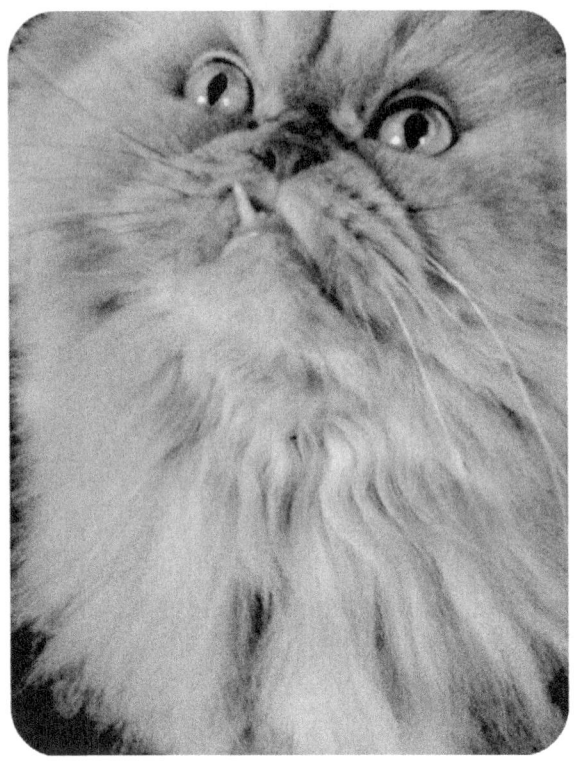

A llergies normally occur when a pet's immune system is overly sensitive to a specific everyday substance, and it can be extremely frustrating for us not knowing what's causing allergy reactions. It may be pollen, dust, an allergic reaction to certain food ingredients, or many other possibilities.

Symptoms:

Symptoms of allergies are; constant sneezing, coughing or wheezing; itchy skin and/or itchy, watery eyes, itchy ears, and possible ear infections. Also, vomiting, diarrhea, sudden snoring caused by an inflamed throat, or chewing of the paws.

Natural Cure/Remedy:

Ginkgo Biloba.

This natural plant extract is a powerful anti-inflammatory, it helps to alleviate bronchial constriction and hyper sensitivity and is best crushed into their food. It is completely safe for animals and higher dosages of Ginkgo Biloba have been given to pets for long period of time without any major side effects.

Use 500 mg of powder/capsule herb per 25-50 of pounds. Use every 8-12 hours or 5-10 drops of tincture per 10 pounds of body weight every 8-12 hours.

This is not recommended for pregnant or lactating cats. Also Ginkgo Biloba should be avoided in pets with impaired blood clotting (whether due to disease or blood-thinning drugs). This natural remedy helps to aid in blood clotting by inhibiting platelet aggregation. Stop giving Ginkgo a week before your cat/dog has to go in for surgery because of the blood thinning properties in this plant can cause complications.

You will be able to find Ginkgo Biloba at health food/herbalist stores.

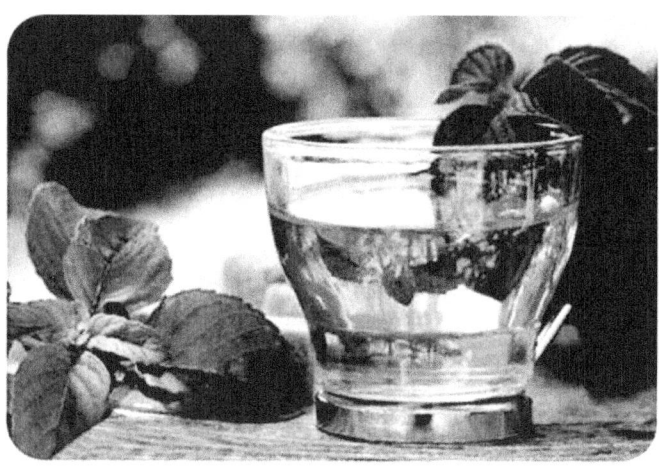

Chamomile:

Applied directly to the skin, concentrated chamomile helps to relieve skin allergies in your pet. It is available in oil infusion, ointment, and as a tea. It may be applied directly to the problem area, or given orally.

For skin irritation add Chamomile flowers to the cat/dogs bath water. These flowers will sooth and heal itchy and problematic skin.

For any eye problems make up a cooled solution and strain with a muslin cloth. Dilute the solution and apply to the infected area several time a day. Chamomile also has anti-inflammatory and antibacterial properties.

If you prefer, you may choose to boil 1 cup of water and make a tea from the chamomile flowers. Allow to brew for 10 - 15 minutes, once cooled, you can place the tea in the pet's water bowl, or soak a treat into the mixture to make it more palatable.

Calendula.

This is a very gentle herb that can help ease skin irritation, rashes, and wounds. It helps to eliminate itchy skin, heals minor wounds, and is also a natural antiseptic.

You may also choose to make a tea solution with Calendula and apply to your pet's eyes and ears. It is available in spray format, gel, as a topical cream, essential oil extract, or tincture.

Calendula is typically found in health food stores and can also be purchased online.

A word of caution. Calendula has the reputation of stimulating early labor contractions of your cat or dog if pregnant.

Licorice Root.

Licorice Root is a natural cortisone. It can be used to soothe allergies and itchy skin in your pet as it holds an anti-inflammatory quality. Apply topically. Licorice tea, salve, or oil infusion, can also be used to relieve skin disorders.

A simple oil infusion Recipe.

What you need:

- Dried licorice root - chopped
- Extra-virgin olive oil

Method:

1. Place the chopped licorice root into a glass jar and cover it sufficiently with olive oil.

2. Leave about a half-inch layer of liquid above the herb.

3. Cover the jar tightly and place it in a warm dark place away from direct sunlight.

4. Store away for one month.

5. Then strain the oil through a sieve, and squeeze what you can from the herb by wrapping it in unbleached muslin or cheesecloth.

6. You will now have sweet-tasting licorice oil that will keep for several months if refrigerated.

7. Apply it topically to your pet's skin as needed.

You will be able to find licorice root at any herbal store.

Organic Apple Cider Vinegar.

This is a wonderful cure for your pets. It improves digestion, boosts the immune system, and gives their coat a beautiful shine. When giving organic apple cider vinegar to your companion, ensure it is unpasteurized and unheated.

Simply mix the apple cider vinegar with equal parts of water in a spray bottle, and Spray directly onto the affected area. Alternatively, you may add a little too unscented wet wipes, or use as a rinse after a bath. You may also add an oral dose mix to a dropper with 1/2tsp per 15lbs of body weight.

Feed your pet a high quality natural food with proper supplements. This will prevent any dietary deficiencies.

Amino Acids: This contains beneficial anti-inflammatory properties and also improves the quality of their skin and coat.

Spoil your pet by brushing their coat regularly. This helps with the even distribution of natural oils.

A natural herbal bath is a gentle alternative to harsh chemicals when getting rid of flees. Wash your pets bedding with hypoallergenic detergent in very hot water.

Homemade Cat Recipes.

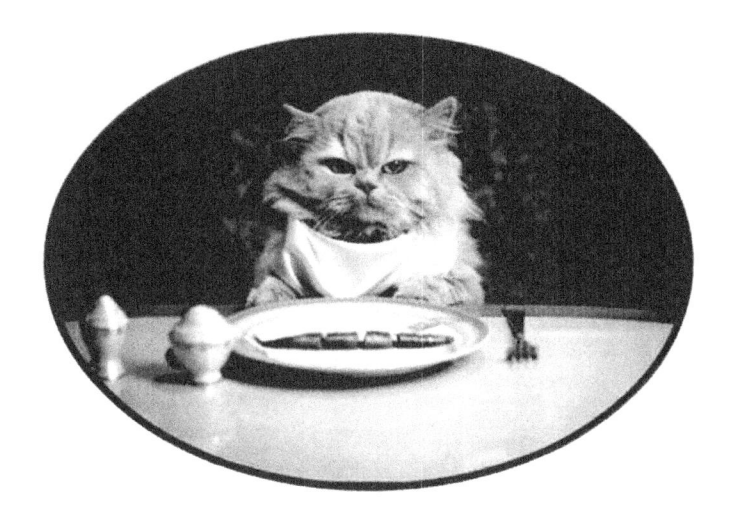

Recent studies suggest that adding a diet that includes correctly boiled raw fowl, or rabbit, may actually help certain cat ailments such as liver and kidney disease. For feline diets, 'raw is gold'. The right balance of ingredients and storage requirements is vital for a jovial and healthy pet. Protein from fish, meat, amino acids, vitamins, water, minerals and fatty acids, are essential for their overall wellbeing. Carbohydrates such as corn and rice may be included in small amounts if your cat doesn't suffer from allergies. Here are a few homemade cat foods that may help treat ailments.

Mackerel Heaven.

- 1 cup of canned mackerel
- 1 tablespoon of sunflower seed oil
- 1 tablespoon of cooked organic brown rice
- 2 tablespoons of beef or chicken broth

Method:

Add all the above ingredients into a food processor and blend on medium, then serve to your cat. Any leftovers can be placed in the fridge using an airtight container. Rice as an ingredient in this dish especially aids cats with sensitive stomachs.

Sardine Recipe:

- 1 can of sardines (with oil)
- 2 tablespoons of grated carrots
- 1/3rd cup of cooked oatmeal

Method:

Mix together and serve. This recipe boosts the immune system and fights inflammation. Sardines contain polyunsaturated fat which also helps cats with kidney disease. This recipe is also great for digestion as it contains no irritable fiber.

Trout Cat Food Recipe:

- 1 cup of cooked trout
- 1 cooked egg yolk
- 1 tablespoon of steamed broccoli
- 2 tbsp. of sunflower oil

Method:

Place all of the ingredients into a food processor, blend on medium, and serve.

The protein in the egg assists in aiding cats with gas, vomiting and diarrhea complications.

Salmon dinner:

- 1 can of salmon
- 1 tablespoon of cooked and mashed broccoli
- ¼ cup of whole wheat bread crumbs
- 1 tablespoon of brewer's yeast

Method:

Combine all the ingredients in a bowl and stir well, then serve. Keep any leftovers refrigerated in an airtight container and discard after three days.

Chicken Dinner:

- 1 cup of cooked chicken
- 1/4 cup of steamed broccoli
- 1/4 cup of steamed carrots
- Chicken broth

Method:

Place all the ingredients into a food processor and puree into a paste. Allow the food to completely cool before serving. Chicken contains polyunsaturated fat which helps treat kidney disease, it also boosts the immune system and reduces inflammation in lymph glands and organ tissue. This dish is also a very good choice for diabetic cats due its high protein content and minimal carbohydrate.

Chicken and Pumpkin Cat Recipe: These ingredients include fresh and boneless organic chicken, freshly steamed pumpkin, grated carrots and mashed sweet potato.

Mince the chicken and then mix with the rest of the pumpkin and vegetables in an 80% to 20% ratio. Roll the mixture into small balls and bake for approximately 25 minutes at a temperature of 170 degrees.

For cats with Inflammatory Bowel Disease (IBD) this recipe presents one of the best choices. This meal is also a transition into a raw and grain free diet.

Beef Dinner:

- 1 cup of ground beef
- 1/2 cup of steamed brown rice
- 6 tablespoons of minced sprouts
- 1 cup of cottage cheese

Method:

Brown the minced beef in a pan and drain it. Allow the beef to cool completely and then mix all the ingredients in a bowl and serve. You may refrigerate the remains for up to three days.

Chicken and Tuna:

- ½ a cup of cooked chicken
- 1 can of tuna (with oil)
- 1 tablespoon of cooked mashed carrot
- 2 tablespoons of brown rice

Method:

Place all ingredients into a food processor and pulse on high until ground. This is ready to serve. Discard any leftovers after three days of refrigeration.

Cat Salad:

- ½ cup of chopped alfalfa sprouts
- ¼ cup of grayed zucchini
- 1 tsp. chicken or fish stock
- 1 small piece of minced catnip

Method:

Combine and toss the first three ingredients into a bowl and sprinkle the catnip on top for garnish. The remaining food can be stored in the refrigerator inside an airtight container for up to three days.

Turkey Balls:

- 1/2 pound of ground turkey
- 1/2 cup of grated carrots
- 1/4 cup of parmesan cheese
- 1 tablespoon of salt
- 1/2 cup of finely crushed crackers
- 1/2 cup of powdered milk
- 1 egg
- 1 tsp. salt
- 1 tbsp. Brewer's yeast

Method:

Preheat the oven to 350 degrees Fahrenheit.

Mix all the ingredients in a large bowl and shape into small balls. Place into the oven for one hour. Let it cool before serving.

Catnip Biscuit Treats:

- 1 1/2 cups of wheat flour
- 1 ½ tsp. catnip
- 1/3 cup of powdered milk
- 1/2 cup of milk
- 1 egg
- 1 tablespoon of honey
- 2 tablespoons of softened butter

Method:

Mix the dry ingredients into a bowl and then slowly add the wet ingredients and mix into a soft dough. Cut the dough into small sized bites and bake for 20 minutes until they are a golden brown. Cool the biscuits and break them apart to serve. Store the remainder in an airtight container or freeze them.

Kitty Bruschetta:

Lightly toast a slice of bread. Cut the toasted bread into small cubes and brush it with canola oil. Sprinkle dry fish flakes onto the bread and bake at 350 degrees F until they achieve a rich golden brown color. Allow the dish to cool slightly and serve while warm.

Cheese Ball Cat Treats:

- 2 tablespoons of margarine
- 1/2 cup of grated cheddar cheese
- 1 egg white
- 1/2 cup of whole wheat flour
- 1/2 teaspoon of dried catnip

Method:

Combine the first three ingredients until well blended. In a separate bowl, combine flour and catnip. Add the flour mixture slowly to the first three ingredients mixing until a soft dough ball is formed. Separate into half-inch pieces and roll by hand into small balls. Place the balls on an ungreased cookie sheet, and bake at 300 degrees F for approximately 25 minutes. This makes approximately twelve balls. Cool completely before serving.

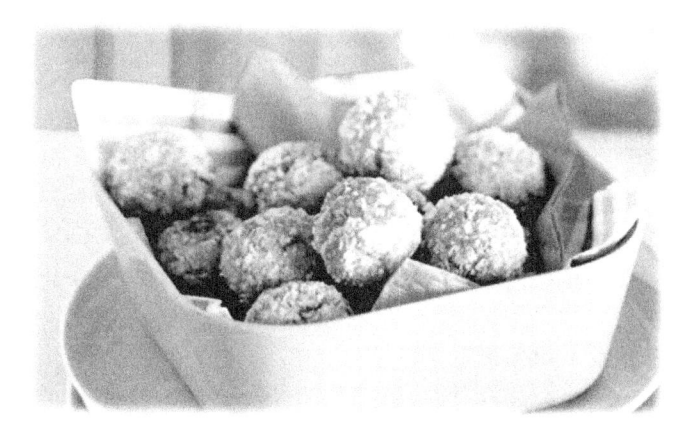

Tuna Ball Jerky Treats:

- 1 cup of whole-wheat flour
- 1/2 cup of powdered milk
- 1/2 cup of tuna packed in oil

- 1 large egg (beaten)
- 1/4 cup of water

Method:

Grease a cookie sheet with margarine. In a bowl, mix the flour and powdered milk together. In a separate bowl, combine the tuna and egg together making sure to mash the tuna in fully. Add the tuna mixture to the dry ingredients, and add the water a little at a time until a slightly sticky dough ball is formed. Roll into balls and place them about one inch apart on a non-stick cookie sheet. Cook in the oven at 350 degrees F for about 25 minutes. Cool completely before serving. Alternatively, you may substitute for cooked, pureed chicken that is mixed with one tablespoon of cod liver oil instead of oiled tuna.

Cat Allergies.

A cat's digestion is very different to our own so don't worry too much about giving them raw meat or fish as long as you boil it first. They have a much shorter intestinal tract. Food and waste passes through their intestines quickly giving less time for bacteria to cause a stomach upset. A properly handled and prepared raw meat and fish diet has much less bacteria in it than many commercial pet foods. Commercial dry cat food may also contain high levels of mold toxins from grains.

Homemade Recipe:

- 32 oz. boneless and skinned chicken thigh (Organic)
- 6 ounces raw liver (Organic)
- 1 8 oz. cup of filtered water, 1 egg (optional)
- 5000 - 10,000mg fish oil (5 - 10 capsules of the average 1000mg capsules)
- 400 IU Vitamin E

- 50mg Vitamin B complex
- 2000mg Taurine Powder
- 5 tsp organic/free range egg shell powder
- 1/2 tsp of Himalayan Salt
- 2 tsp Psyllium Husk
- 3 tsp Unflavored Gelatin

Method:

Chop half of the chicken thigh meat and liver into about half inch chunks. This is important for their dental health. Grind the other remaining half of the meat in a grinder or food processor. Mix the grinded meat in with the meat chunks. In a separate bowl, mix all the remaining ingredients together until smooth. Add this to the meat and mix well. Divide the mixture up into separate meals, and place in the refrigerator. The serving size will be one cup per day.

Dental Health.

Toothpaste made with Aloe Vera and Bee Propolis:

Both Aloe Vera and Bee Propolis have wonderful healing properties. Propolis is a resinous substance that is collected by honey bees and used to varnish honey combs. Together, they have a healthful effect in treating mouth ailments from bad breath to gingivitis. Bee Propolis is used for its extra antibacterial and immune boosting qualities.

Brown Rice: Bad digestion can play a role in bad breath. Try adding cooked brown rice to your cat/dogs meals.

Parsley and Sage spray: Make your own mouth spray by making a tea. Add a few sprigs of parsley and sage into hot water. Once it has cooled, strain the tea and put in a spray bottle. Spritz this mixture in your pet's mouth. Parsley will help freshen their breath, and sage is a natural antiseptic.

Bladder Problems.

Bladder ailments occur mainly in male cats. If left untreated, your pet runs the risk of blockage of the Urethra. If this happens, it can cost you a lot of money if taken to the vet to get it seen too.

Here are a few natural remedies to help your kitty with bladder and kidney issues.

Nature Remedy Cranberries: If your cat has a bladder infection (UTI), cranberries can be a wonderful and natural cure for a healthy bladder and kidney system. Used on a regularly basis, cranberries can prevent bacteria causing infection. If your cat or dog had bladder problems in the past the chances are that they may get it again. Prevention is always key. Here are a few ways to use cranberries in your pet's diet.

Unsweetened cranberry juice: This is an old natural remedy that will always come to the rescue. Cranberry increases urine acidity which lessens the risk of blockages or infections within the body. It also prevents bacteria from sticking to the bladder walls. Try mixing a little cranberry juice with their water.

Gel Capsule: Cranberry extract 1/8 capsule for cats & small dogs, 1/4 capsule for medium dogs, 1/2 capsule for large dogs. This should be given three times per day for a total of 3-5 days, or until symptoms subside.

Homemade tasty treats for bladder problems:

- 2 organic eggs
- 1/2 organic extra virgin olive oil
- 1 cup organic pumpkin puree
- 1 1/2 organic cups oats or your choice of whole grain flour
- 1 1/2 teaspoons organic cinnamon
- 1 teaspoon organic carob powder
- 1 teaspoon baking soda
- 1 teaspoon baking powder
- 1/2 teaspoon sea salt
- 1/2 cup organic dried cranberries finely chopped

Method:

Preheat oven to 375F degrees. Whisk the eggs, oil, and pumpkin puree in a food processor. In a separate bowl, add all the dry ingredients and mix well. Add the dry ingredients to the wet ingredients and blend until smooth. Fold in the chopped cranberries. Line a mini muffin pan with paper cups, and fill each cup with the muffin mixture. Bake in the preheated oven for about 15 minutes. Remove muffins from oven and cool completely. Store in an airtight container.

Feed your cat with a high quality all natural wet food.

Dry foods have low moisture content. Cats get most of their water from the food they eat. If your cat is eating only dry foods, it could be they are not getting sufficient water which may lead to bladder and kidney problems.

Vitamin C:

When you notice that your dog/cat is having bladder problems. Ensure your cat gets a daily dose of between 250 - 500mg of Vitamin C every day. Vitamin C is a natural anti-inflammatory. This will aid in a painful, irritated and inflamed bladder to heal itself.

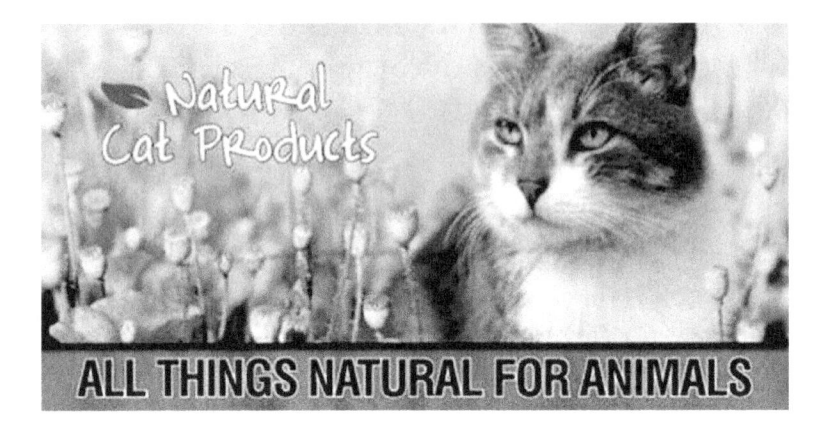

Herbal Remedies.

Bear's grape is a strong diuretic which kills bacteria within the bladder. It also supports the urinary tract system. The leaves are impervious to water so making tea with the leaves will be almost impossible. Take one cup of herbs and add 3 cups of water. Allow for it to cool. Give one teaspoon of herbs to the pet once per day and do not exceed more than 3 days. Administer in their water dish, food, or by using a syringe.

Oregon grape holly contains a natural antibiotic. This helps to kill strep and staph bacteria. It can also alleviate symptoms of an inflamed bladder. These dried herb leaves are available at any herbal/health store.

Lyceum is used as a traditional remedy for many different ailments. It is rich in amino acids and it nourishes the liver and kidneys.

Cats with Colds and Flu Symptoms.

Just like ourselves, cats are not immune to colds and the flu. The symptoms are; sneezing, red or swollen eyes, discharge from the nose and/or eyes, lack of appetite, and mobility issues. This can last for about 7 - 14 days depending on how bad the virus infection is.

The best thing you can do is to make your cat as comfortable as possible. Ensure they are kept warm and have a comfy spot to sleep. If there is discharge from eyes/nose, swab the area with a mild saline mixture. Make the solution with one teaspoon of salt and 450ml of warm water.

Keep the room well ventilated. Make sure there is sufficient clean water and encourage your cat to drink often. Put food, water and litter close to where your pet is sleeping. They will have joint pain and won't be able to move around much. Give them a strong smelling fish like pilchards or sardines. This will encourage them to eat because of a reduced sense of smell. If they have very little appetite, try giving them full cream ice cream. This will also help soothe their sore throat. Keep other cats away as cat flu is extremely contagious and make their surrounding environment stress free.

Echinacea boosts the immune system. Preferably use sweet Echinacea used for children. It is alcohol free. Give the sick kitty 1/2 a child's dose, 2 times per day for about 7 days. For dogs, give them a powdered form. It has been suggested to give dogs 45mg/lb. of body weight once a day. Echinacea is readily available at any health store, or pharmacy.

Vitamin C can also work well as it is contains antioxidant and antiviral properties.

Ascorbate Acid. Never give this to your pet. This will aggravate their stomach. It's best to use Sodium Ascorbate Crystals and administer about 250mg once per day for a week. If they get an upset stomach, cut back on the dosage.

Colloidal Silver: This kills many different bacterial ailments and is a wonderful alternative to antibiotics. Use about one third of the recommended dosage that we ourselves take three times a day for about a week. You can also wipe the cat's eyes, nose and ears with colloidal silver.

Bee Propolis has been used throughout history as a natural remedy to fight off germs. It heals wounds, tumors and abscesses. It is a natural antibiotic, anti-viral, and also has anti-parasitic properties. Give them 1/4 of the dosage recommended for human consumption. Administer the dosage to your pet about 4 times per day until the symptoms subside.

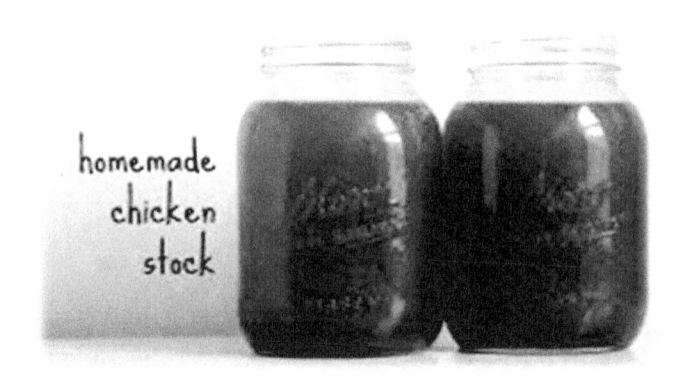

Chicken stock for Sick Cats:

- 1 organic chicken thigh
- Add a few fresh sprigs of sage, rosemary and parsley,
- add a vegetable of your choice such as carrot

Method:

1. Mix all the ingredients in a pot of water and allow to simmer on low heat.

2. After about 3 hours of simmering, let the soup cool.

3. Remove the bones from the meat and cut the meat finely.

4. Remove the vegetables and herbs.

5. Do not skim the fat off from the liquid.

6. Place in a bowl and encourage your sick pet to drink the broth. Give this to them about 3 times a day or until symptoms lesson.

Cats, Head to Paw.

Anxious and Restless Cats.

Essential oils have been used for hundreds of years, not only for ourselves but for our animals. For anxious or restless cats, try adding a few drops of lavender oil to a small handkerchief and tie loosely around your cat's collar. Be sure to use a carrier oil, as pure essential oils are highly concentrated and can irritate their skin.

Fractionated coconut oil, diluted to about 20% (that's 2 drops of lavender oil and 8 drops of coconut oil). You can also put a few drops of this diluted mixture on the inside of his/her collar.

Lavender oil can be dispersed within your home through an aromatherapy diffuser. It has the ability to calm and soothe. Essential oils and fractionated coconut oil can be found at most specialty food stores.

Watery eyes. A cat's eyes should be bright and clear. If you notice your cat is pawing at his/her eyes, wiping them on the couch or carpet, or they have a gooey film around them, it could be an indication of allergies. First, wipe your cat's eyes with a warm, damp cloth. Use a weak hydrogen peroxide mixture to cleanse around the eyes being careful not to get any hydrogen peroxide into them. You can also use all natural eye drops that can be found through holistic pet stores. Treat aching eyes with a warm, chamomile tea bag. Be sure it is not too hot, as eyes are a very sensitive part of the body. If the problem persists, or worsens, this could be a more serious bacterial infection, and you should consider seeking guidance with your local vet.

Cat acne. Have you ever been scratching underneath your cat's chin and found tiny, black flecks on your fingertips? You may have thought these were flea eggs or dirt, but it may be acne tissue. Cat acne cannot be cured, but is easily managed and treated with some diligence. Avoid plastic food and water bowls in case an allergic reaction is to blame. Plastic dishes are also a magnet for germs and bacteria. Opt in for ceramic or glass dishes. Check and refresh your cat's water regularly (1-2 times a day) to be sure these little bacterial issues stay away from your cat's furry face. The infection usually responds well to cleansing of the skin twice daily with an ointment or gel containing 2.5 to 5 percent benzoyl peroxide, chlorhexidine (Nolvasan) or Betadine. Epson salts will promote drainage to the area, and Aloe Vera may soothe it. Further steps, including topical medication may be necessary, but try these easy home remedies to treat mild cases.

Hairballs may be an indication of poor pet grooming. As much as we like to believe that cats have great hygiene, sometimes they need a little help. Groom your cat regularly by brushing him/her once daily with a high quality, undercoat comb. This will pull out the clotted, often harder to reach fur that is ailing your pet. You may be surprised how much of a difference it makes in the look and feel of their fur. Regular combing releases natural oils within their skin to the surface layers. This in turn makes the coat silky and healthier in appearance. You may want to occasionally wipe him/her down with a damp towel to take away any residual dirt and dander.

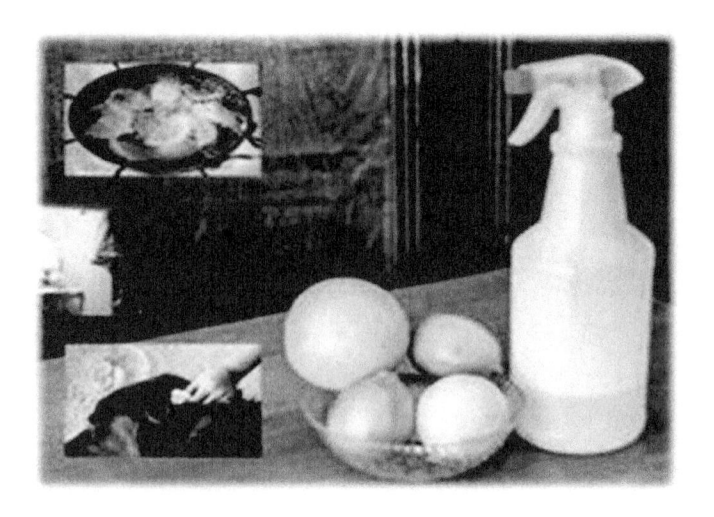

Natural Remedies for your furry friends.

Make the Flea's Flee!

The love and investment that goes into keeping our pets sound and healthy is not so difficult if we know what to do. Here we will be focusing on some natural cures for ailments in pets concerning fleas and its negative effects on your pet. There are many benefits to homeopathic remedies that don't require poison to kill these little pests.

All Natural flea and Tick Remedies:

Essential oils are used often by humans to treat everything from anxiety to decreased energy. Luckily, fleas and ticks are not major problems for us, but they are for our pets. One of the easiest tick remedies is **rose geranium essential oil**. Apply a few drops to your pet's collar to repel these nasty guys. Fleas are just as annoying and possibly more dangerous as many pets have allergies to flea bites causing major itching, rough scratching, and rashes. Below are more home remedies you can try at home.

The Magic of the Chamomile Tea: This can be sprayed or applied topically, due to its rich herbal extracts, it can solve not only flea infestations, but also aid any eye inflammation and stomach irritation.

Method:

Place four Chamomile tea bags into boiling water and let them steep for 15 minutes before cooling. Rinse the affected area with the cooled tea. You can also apply it directly using a cloth or a spray bottle. Store the remainder of the tea in an air tight container and place in the fridge. You can use this solution for up to three days.

Step up the game: You can give your pet a good start by putting a little garlic and Brewer's Yeast in your dog's food. This singular diet keeps flea's away, and prevents itching and discomfort. However, it must be stated that garlic is not good for cats.

Flea Combs: Most over-the-counter and vet flea medication contains poison. When a pet consumes these medications orally, the poison works through the system and secretes into the outer skin layer, thus, killing fleas and larvae. Flea combs can be time consuming but they are none toxic and safe to use.

The Beauty of Oil: Neem Oil and Coconut oil are a great way to keep the fleas at bay. This is due to the rich elements derived from them. You should use coconut oil in small quantities due to its strong and pungent abilities.

Keep it juicy and healthy: Another good preventive measure is apply fresh orange or lemon juice topically to your pet as fleas do not like citrus.

The Collar of your pet can be a great help. Rose Geranium oil when dabbed onto their collar can help keep fleas away.

Oatmeal can also do the trick: Mix the oatmeal to a paste using a little water. Let it work its magic for 10 minutes, then wash it off.

Aloe Vera is extremely effective in tackling many issues of the skin that affect your pets, including fleas. Apply it topically but care must be taken to ensure that your pets do not ingest this substance as it has a strong laxative effect. Aloe Vera contains nutrients that make it ideal for soothing healing/itching wounds, or sores from flea bites.

Flea Repellent. Many store bought flea repellents contain toxic chemicals that may make your pet's skin and fur dry and itchy. Cats tend to groom themselves often which increase their likelihood of ingesting the chemicals.

Make a batch of your own homemade flea repellent.

What you need:

- 3-5oz squirt bottle
- 2 cups water
- 1 large sliced lemon
- 1 handful of fresh lavender sprigs (or 1 tbsp. of dried lavender)
- 2 tsp. alcohol free witch hazel

Method:

1. Place the water, lemon slices, and lavender sprigs in a small saucepan and simmer for about 20-30 minutes.

2. Remove from the heat to cool. The water should be a light purple-pink color.

3. Once cooled, pour the mixture through a fine mesh sieve, reserving the liquid in a small bowl. You can throw out the lavender sprigs and lemon slices when done.

4. Pour the liquid into a small squirt bottle and add a sprig or two of lavender to keep the solution smelling fresh.

To Use:

Apply a few squirts onto your cat's back and rub into his/her fur. One bottle usually lasts 1-2 weeks.

Flea and tick repellent.
What you need:

- 8 oz. Apple cider vinegar
- 4 oz. warm water
- 1/2 tsp salt
- 1/2 tsp baking soda

Method:

1. Mix salt and baking soda in to a small dish, then mix vinegar and water in a separate dish.

2. Slowly add the dry ingredients to the wet ingredients (vinegar may react slightly to baking soda but this is normal)

3. Add to a medium spray bottle and spray onto your pet.

Note: You can also sprinkle borax on the carpets in your home, and vacuum. This will help combat any fleas or flea eggs that may still be in your carpet.

Oil of lemon Eucalyptus to Deter Mosquitos:

This plant derived compound is an effective remedy for repelling mosquitoes. This compound can work for up to four to six hours depending on several factors including how much the wearer perspires. Commonly called 'lemon eucalyptus', the repellent is readily available in spray format, or as an essential oil. Dab a little amount on to the outside of their collar.

Prevent Ticks:

Garlic given as a dietary supplement makes your dog or cat less appealing to ticks. The aroma is excreted through the skin and repels both ticks and fleas. However, garlic contain sulfoxides and disulfides, which can damage red blood cells and cause anemia in pets. If you use garlic as a tick prevention, use it sparingly.

Apple Cider Vinegar. Apple cider vinegar adds acidity to your pet's blood stream making it less appealing to ticks and fleas. Add 2 tablespoons of the apple cider vinegar to your pet's food or water bowl as a preventative measure.

Kidney Health:

Some cats, especially male cats are prone to blockages in the bladder and urinary tract system.

You may administer orally ¼ of a gel cranberry supplement capsule once daily, or add a splash of 100% cranberry juice into their water. Cranberry decreases the likelihood of any issues by increasing the acidity of the urine.

Tummy Troubles: Pets who may have been prescribed antibiotics recently, may develop stomach issues and discomfort since antibiotics wipe out good bacteria that naturally resides in the stomach. To counteract this, give your pet a little natural yogurt with their evening meal to help boost the re growth of beneficial bacteria within their system. Be sure to choose a yogurt that is free of flavored varieties because of its added preservatives and high sugar content. Mix in with their food.

Diarrhea: It is often recommended that you refrain from feeding your pet for 24 hours if he/she is suffering from diarrhea. It is likely something they have ate that is contributing to this ailment. Doing this will flush out any toxins. Provide plenty of water to avoid dehydration since diarrhea can be taxing on your pet's body. When your pet does start eating again, keep it bland. To help solidify the stool, try a teaspoon or two of canned pumpkin. This fibrous squash can help rectify diarrhea. Although cats are lactose intolerant, milk will also help this ailment. You can also dilute 20 drops of slippery elm tincture in to 1 oz. of spring water. Give this to your cat orally via a small dropper up to three times a day until symptoms decrease.

Weight Loss

Cat Body Condition Chart.

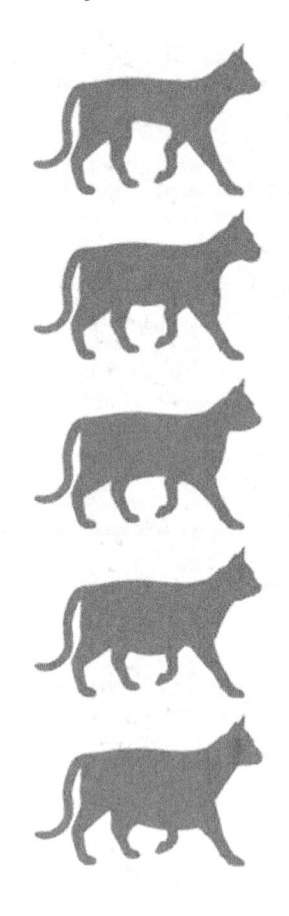

Thin
Protruding pelvic bones
Narrow waist
Pronounced tuck in the abdomen
Extremely bony and weak

Underweight
Ribs and vertebrae visible
Tapered waist
Slight tuck in the abdomen
Lean and skinny

Ideal
Bones not visible, but can be felt
Muscular waist
Raised abdomen, no sagging
Healthy and muscular

Overweight
Bones hidden under fat
Fuller waist
Sagged abdomen
Stout appearance

Obese
Extremely chubby body
Rolls of fat around waist and neck
Distended, sagged abdomen
Very bulky appearance

Exercise: We all know that the key to weight loss is exercise, and it is the same for animals too. But, few of us envision taking our cats for walks outside on a harness and leash. If you prefer not to use this method, carefully select a few cat toys that will help even the older adult cats feel young again. The key is to select interactive toys and treat toys.

Laser pointers are great for getting your cat's juices flowing, or additionally, select a toy that has something that he/she can catch such as 'The Birdie'. Think feather on a string. Continue active play until your cat is panting, then let your cat win and revel in their successful hunt.

Scratch posts: Cats are natural hunters and to keep their claws sharp. There are many modern and sleek designs to choose from that are attractive in design. This addition to your home will give your cat something to scratch on that isn't your couch.

Muscle aches: Use Epsom salts to treat strains and sprains. Dissolve some Epsom salts in hot water, let the water cool and then soak a wash cloth into the mixture. Apply this to the area, and let it absorb into their skin.

N P A: Nutrition, **P**lay time, and **A**ffection, are three of the most important aspects of keeping your feline happy and healthy. Select wholesome, grain free cat food to help improve their health. Stay away from ingredients that may not occur naturally in a cat's diet. Look for high sources of protein and allergy free food. Ironically, many felines are allergic to fish and fish products. If a particular food brand does not list fish, or states it is gluten-free, then it is likely a good diet. If a label says it is all natural then go for it! Ingredients that are listed as all natural have had no chemical alterations made to it.

Homemade Tuna Cat Treats:

What you need:

- 1 4 oz. can of tuna in water
- 1/4 Cup tuna water (if needed, top off with tap water to make 1/4 cup)
- 2 egg whites, cooked and roughly chopped
- 1/4 cup corn meal

- 1/4 cup whole wheat flour

Method:

1. Use a food processor on medium and pulse the tuna and egg whites until fine. Add water and continue blending.

2. Add corn meal and whole wheat flour and pulse until well combined. The mixture should form a dough like consistency.

3. Lightly flour your work space, and roll out the dough until it is approximately 1/4 inch thick. Using a knife to cut the dough into small rectangles (about 1/2 inch each).

4. Place each treat on a lightly greased baking sheet and bake at 350 degrees Fahrenheit for about 15-18 minutes or until lightly browned.

5. Allow to cool to room temperature and store in an airtight container.

These treats will keep in the refrigerator for up to 7 days, or you may freeze them for up to 3 months.

DIY Cat Toy

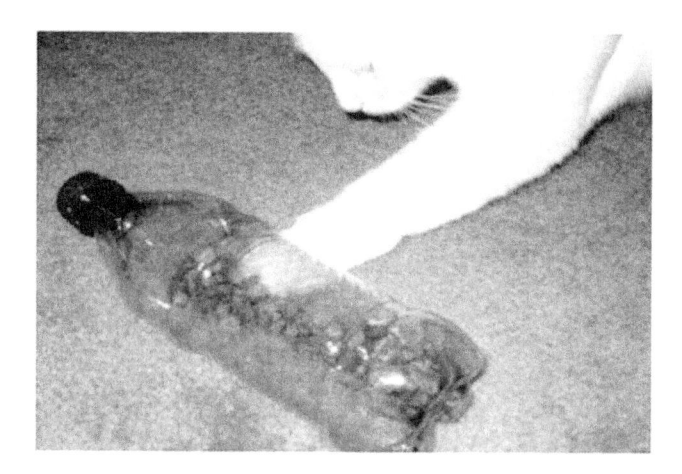

You will need an empty water bottle. Cut a few small holes into it and place cat treats inside. The more your frisky feline bats this homemade toy around, the more treats he/she will get! Take it up a notch by filling it with the homemade tuna treats listed above.

Grocery Shopping List for Cats

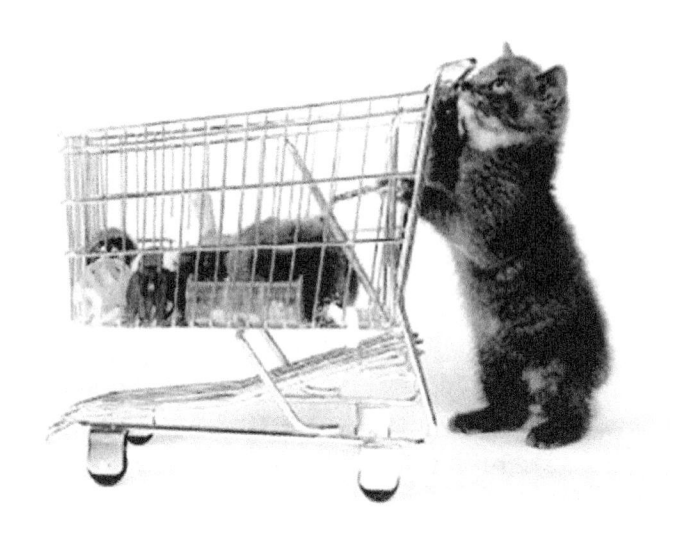

Meat.

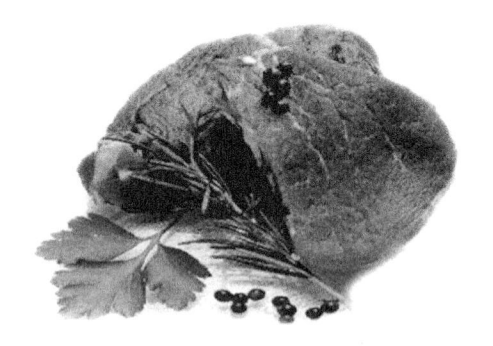

Whole Chicken
Chicken breast/thighs
Ground Beef
Ground Turkey

Produce.

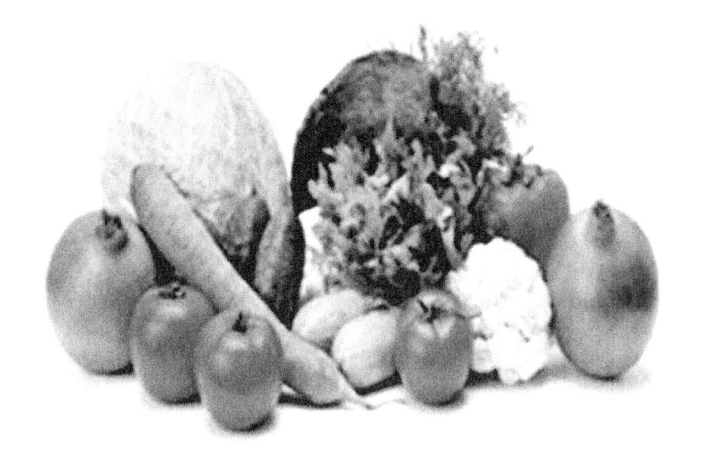

Broccoli
Carrots
Sweet potatoes
Zucchini
Pumpkin
Dried Cranberries
Parsley/Sage/Rosemary

Poultry.

Eggs
Cottage cheese
Parmesan cheese/cheddar
Powdered milk
Tuna
Sardines/Bream
Salmon
Mackerel
Trout
Liver

Grains/Nuts/Other.

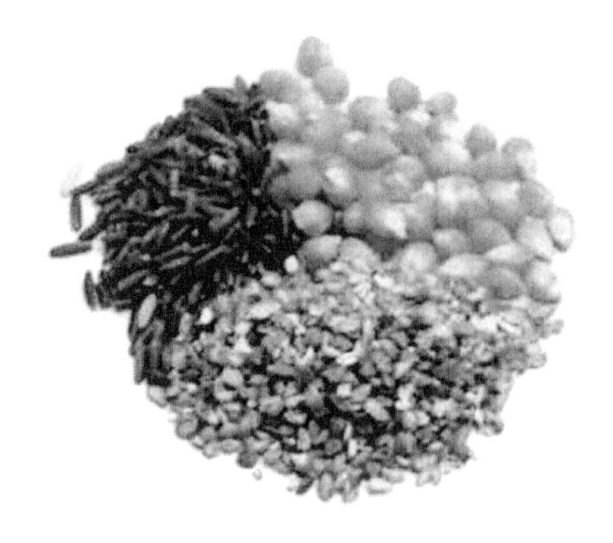

Whole Wheat Bread
Wheat/whole grain Flour
Crackers
Sun flower oil
Canola oil
Brewer's yeast
Oatmeal
Brown rice
Minced sprouts
Alfalfa sprouts
Salt
Honey
Butter/margarine
Cinnamon
Minced catnip
Carob powder
Fish flakes
Egg shell powder
Taurine powder

Husk
Gelatin (unflavored)
Psyllium
Vitamin B complex/Vitamin E

Pets and Tapeworms.

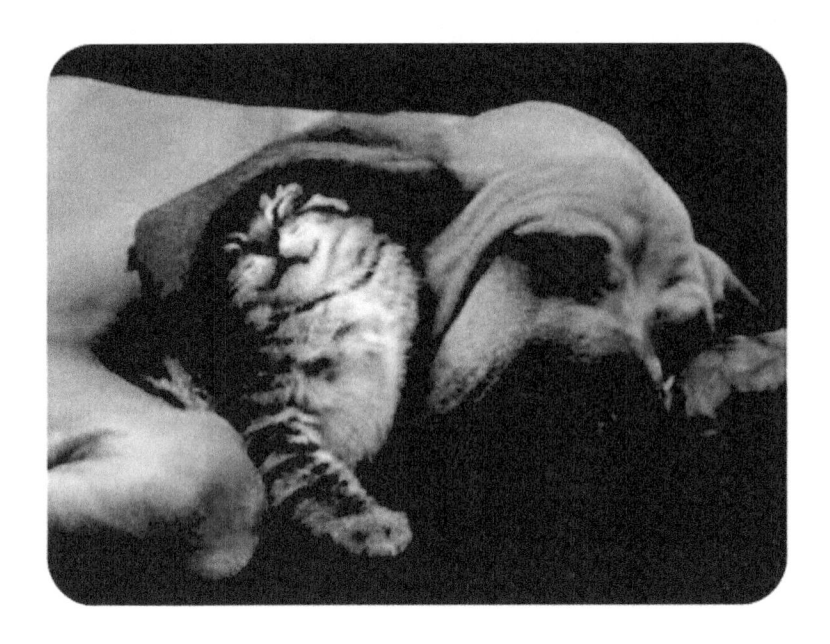

Natural remedies using Homeopathy

When it comes to treating tapeworms at home, there are many options using natural remedies.

Pumpkin seeds are a great way to help get rid of tapeworms. You simply need to grind them up and give to your pet with their meal. For every 10 lbs. mix in a teaspoon of the ground pumpkin seed. Not only does it fight to rid the body of worms, but it is also a great supplement to add to their diet.

A tincture of **Oregon grape** also works well to treat worms.

Wheat germ oil is also a good way to help prevent an infestation.

Garlic is another way to expel tapeworms. Feeding fresh or powdered garlic daily to your pet, can rid them of tapeworms in approximately two months. Tapeworms do not particularly like the sulfur compound in garlic. For dogs, use 1/2 to 1 whole clove daily and for cats, 1/4 to 1/2 clove.

Cloves in small amounts, can also rid your pet of tapeworms. It contains anti-parasitic, antiseptic, and antibacterial properties. By giving one clove daily, after meals, for a week should help with the worms.

Wormwood oil and olive oil mixed together, is another natural remedy for treating tapeworms. Mix one part wormwood oil and eight parts olive oil. A teaspoon for a large dog and two drops for puppy's, small dogs, and cats.

Fennel is a great herb for expelling tapeworms, and also helps to strengthen your pet's immune system.

Carrot (grinded) works well if adding it to your pet's food. This serves as a preventative measure with fighting worms. Carrot also helps keep the digestive tract clean.

Parsley: A simple recipe for parsley is grinding it and then cooking it in water for three minutes. Strain the mixture, and pour it into an ice cube tray. Freeze it then pop a cube out and give it to your dog at meal time.

Diatomaceous works well for the treatment of worms. It is commercially made, but is an all-natural product. The dosage for Diatomaceous is as follows:

For kittens use 1/2 teaspoon, for adult cats use 1 teaspoon, small dogs 1/2 teaspoon, 2 teaspoons for dogs under 50 lbs. and large dog breeds over 50 lbs. 1 tablespoon.

Cayenne pepper (dried) Adding this to food can eliminate tapeworms and it may also aid in preventing future infestations.

Apple cider vinegar is another great way to rid your dogs of tapeworms. It is readily available, and just 1 teaspoon given daily to your pet is all that is needed until symptoms subside. Sometimes just being more aware of your pets diet can help a great deal in treating and preventing worm infestation. Worms like a diet rich in sugar and fat. It is best to avoid these while treating your pet for worms as it can make the expulsion of worms harder to beat.

Probiotics eat away the outer layer of worms until they release their hold on the intestinal wall. Probiotics are naturally found in plain yogurt and can be fed to your pet daily.

Acidophilus rebuilds regular intestinal flora. Give your pet one capsule daily.

Recipes

Supplement Recipe: An anti-worm recipe using natural ingredients can make tapeworm treatment more beneficial.

- 2 part raw, ground pumpkin seed
- 1 part garlic powder
- 1 part fennel seed
- 1 part yucca root

Mix all the ingredients together and give daily one teaspoon per pound of pet food.

Simple recipes using fruit can also help in the treatment of tapeworms. By adding grated **coconut** and **papaya** to food can make the intestinal tract much less appealing to tapeworms. **Pineapple** is another fruit that can kill tapeworms. Pineapple contains a digestive enzyme called bromelain that clears the digestive tract of such parasites.

Black walnut is extremely effective is ridding the body of parasites but it also contains a laxative effect so care must be taken if giving this to your pet. Compounds in this herb infuse the blood with more oxygen which, in turn, kills the parasites.

Parsley water is a simple way to help rid the body of tapeworms. Here's how you make it.

Bring 1 quart of water to a boil, add one bunch of fresh parsley and simmer for three minutes. After it has simmered, remove from heat and let cool. Remove and toss out the parsley. Pour the water into a glass jar, and put it in the refrigerator. The dosage is one tablespoon per every 10 lbs. of body weight. Administer once per day for ten days straight. Most de-wormer treatments are given for ten days.

Many of these ingredients are used for more than one ailment which makes them an excellent, safe, and cost effective choice in treating your cats and dogs. The health benefits are abundant and the side-effects minimal.

Home Treatments for Dental Health.

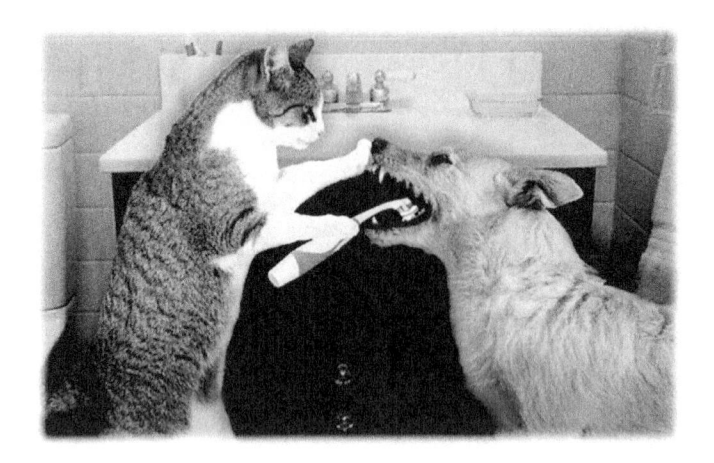

A basic and simple way to clean your pet's teeth is to use a wash cloth, or gauze with water. Simply soak the cloth or gauze in water and wipe out their mouths by gently rubbing their teeth and gums. Do this once daily. This simple method works by removing any food debris left on the teeth before it can sit and cause any gum problems. The best method for treating gingivitis is prevention. There are a number of things you can do at home to keep your pets mouth healthy and free of bacteria. Giving your dog or cat raw bones to chew on is an excellent method of helping to keep your pet's teeth clean. The chewing action scrapes along the teeth and especially along the gum line. This is a great home remedy for cat owners as cats can be a tad more difficult to accept teeth brushing.

Coconut oil toothpaste: Simply dip the toothbrush (or gauze) into the oil and use it to brush their teeth. Another good use of coconut oil is to soak an antler chew in it, and let your pet chew away, this works well with dogs, but some cats enjoy this too.

Method

- 1/2 teaspoon of kelp
- 1/8 tablespoon of parsley flakes
- 1 cup of coconut oil
- 1/2 teaspoon of turmeric

Mix all ingredients in with the oil, store in an airtight container and place it in the fridge. You may have to warm the oil in hot water to mix well. This is 100% organic, so no need to worry if your pet decided to swallow some as you're brushing their teeth.

Mouth Wash or Spray:

These recipes below are pretty simple and straight forward. You may use peppermint oil, spearmint oil, and cinnamon oil for this recipe using one drop of each. Add the oils to distilled water, only about 5 or so milliliters, then place in a small spray bottle and you have a nice mouth wash spray.

If you prefer, you can also add this recipe to their bowl of drinking water. These essential oils are good for their breath, but more importantly, by rinsing out their mouths, it helps to keep any food debris down and that means less bacteria to form along the gum line which is where gingivitis begins.

Herbal Tea:

You may use parsley and mint for this tea and add catnip as well. This works especially well for felines.

Method

Boil water, add the tea bag or dried herbs, and steep for 3-5 minutes. Pour into a glass jar or similar container, and place in the fridge too cool down. Once cooled, either pour approximately 1/4 of tea into their water bowl, or pour some in a spray bottle and use it as a mouth wash. If your pet doesn't like the mint flavor, you may choose not to include that, and just use parsley as this herb is not as strong.

Lemon water is another option to use as a mouthwash.

Liquid Chlorophyll. By just placing a few drops into their water bowls will help with the health of their teeth and gums. Chlorophyll is exceptionally good for fighting off disease including gum disease. It also comes in a dried form that you can crush and sprinkle on top of your pet's food or add to their water dish.

Fruits and vegetables can help with home dental care for your dog. Raw vegetables and fruits are an excellent choice as a snack for them as they are low in fat and crunching away on these veggies help keep their teeth clean. Celery, carrots, apples, and watermelon make good choices. Simply slice them up and give as a treat.

Freezing carrots or watermelon are a good choice for cooling your dog's gums. With the kitties, it is best to cook and dice up the veggies which makes these vegetables more palatable and easier to chew. Adding Cilantro and parsley to food can aid in keeping their breath fresh.

Homemade Healthy Dental Treats:

Try making a batch of homemade dog biscuits and cat chews using cinnamon. Cinnamon can help improve bad breath and biscuits help scrape tartar off teeth.

You can make your own dental treats at home for your dog or cat. Here's a recipe for dogs:

- 3 1/2 cups Brown rice flour
- 1 tablespoon Charcoal
- 4 tablespoons vegetable oil
- 1 Egg
- ½ cup Mint
- ½ to 1 cup Parsley Broth or Water
- Chlorophyll (liquid form)

Method:

Preheat your oven to 400 degrees. Combine the flour and charcoal, and set aside for now. Combine the mint, parsley, oil, and 1/4 of the broth and/or water into a blender or food processor. Blend together finely and add approximately one teaspoon of the chlorophyll. Add this to the flour and charcoal and mix together. Beat the egg and add that in. Knead and add in the remaining broth and/or water. Roll it out and cut out. Bake for 15-20 minutes. You'll definitely want these on the crunchy side as that is partly why they are dental treats. The firm and crunchiness of the texture help scrape any tarter build up.

Tuna fish Cat Treat:

- 1 can Tuna (drained)
- Flour (1 cup) Flour
- 1 cup Cornmeal
- 1/2 cup Parsley
- 1/4 cup Mint
- 1/4 cup Catnip
- 1/3 cup Water

Method:

Preheat the oven to 350 degrees. Hand mix all the ingredients together. Make sure you are using the dried version of the herbs versus fresh as it mixes easier. If you use fresh herbs, just be sure that it is chopped up fine. Roll the dough into the thickness you prefer, and cut into strips. Then cut the strips until you have a treat the size of a dry cat food piece. Bake for about 20 minutes or until nice and crunchy.

Just as with the dog treats, crunchier is better.

The Holistic Approach to Dog Ailments.

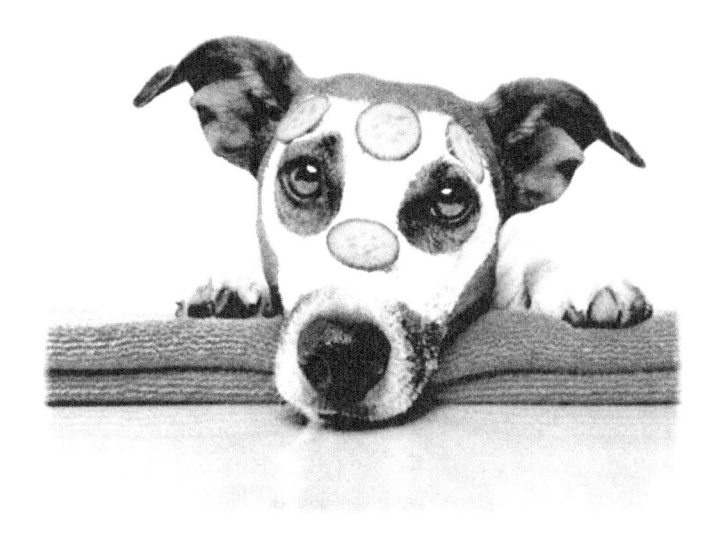

As pet owners, we hate it when our pets aren't feeling at their best. A number of minor ailments can cause your dog to feel under the weather. Try these all natural, home remedies to give your furry friend the best possible holistic care and also keep some money in your pocket. The natural approach to canine health can save you hundreds of dollars per year by avoiding costly vet visits. As always, consult a veterinarian if your dog's symptoms increase in frequency or severity. For minor aches and pains, use these ideas to treat your pet the natural way.

Dry or Cracked Nose: While it is true that a dry, hot nose can be a sign of fever, it is also quite common for a dogs nose to become dry or cracked without any serious illness. For instance, dry air, overexposure to sun, or wind may all be reasons for a dry nose. Simply wash your dog's nose with warm water and soap, avoiding harsh, overly scented soaps which can exacerbate the issue. Then apply a small amount of petroleum jelly to his/her nose. Provide plenty of water to help counteract any possible dehydration.

Ear Infection: A nasty ear infection can be problematic for your canine friend. To treat this ailment in its beginning stages, use **almond oil**. Apply with an ear dropper to administer a teaspoon of warm almond oil in each ear. This will help loosen any wax accumulation and prevent a more serious infection.

A simple, warm compress around the ears can help ease irritation, inflammation, and minor aches and pains. Take this up a notch by cleansing his/her ears with an apple **cider vinegar** solution. Dilute 2 tablespoons of apple cider vinegar in one cup of water. Apply this to your dog orally or use it as a cleansing solution around the ears in combination with the warm compress. If antibiotics are needed, please consult your veterinarian.

Itchy and Watery Eyes: A clear, watery discharge coming from your dog's eyes could be a sign of allergies. If these are seasonal allergies, use a simple home remedy to ease the discomfort. For more serious allergies, consult your vet for possible causes and treatment options. Clean away any discharge with a warm compress. Do this several times daily for best results. If problems persist, use a homemade saline solution by combining a teaspoon of non-iodized salt with 1 cup of distilled water. Rinse your dog's eyes out with this solution twice daily.

Poison Treatment:

As soon as you think your pet has been poisoned you should take him/her to the vet immediately. If you are unable to do so, here are a few tips that can come in useful:

Activated charcoal can be given orally with a large syringe or with a stomach tube. Activated charcoal should not be given to animals that have ingested caustic materials. It should be noted, that those substances that are only slightly adsorbed by charcoal in humans, are likewise poorly adsorbed in your pets. The recommended dose of activated charcoal for animals is 1-3 gm of charcoal per 1 kg body weight. Repeated doses of activated charcoal every four to eight hours at half the original dose may be indicated when there is a possibility of reabsorption of poisons filtered out by the liver. There are many forms of poison for our pets which should be avoided, these include; chocolate, grapes, raisins, fertilizer, household plants, pest bait, cocoa bean mulch, alcohol, nuts, mothballs, fabric softener, antifreeze, the list goes on. Please keep all hazardous materials far from the reach of your pet.

Hydrogen peroxide will help to induce vomiting. Administer one teaspoon per five pounds of weight, and watch carefully. Consult a vet immediately if symptoms do not markedly improved. To improve overall gut function and balance, treat your pet with some plain Greek yogurt.

Symptoms of your pet being poisoned may include vomiting, blood coming from their mouth or stool, lethargy, diarrhea, or seizures.

Poison can also cause liver damage or internal bleeding especially if not treated immediately.

Ear Mites:

Using a herbal stringent made from **yellow dock**, otherwise known as Rumex Crispus, will rid the ears of ear mites. Use 3 drops of yellow dock tincture, and 1 tablespoon of distilled or filtered water. Dilute yellow dock tincture in the water. Instill

1/2 of a dropper full in to the ear canal and massage gently. Let the animal shake its head, then blot with cotton swabs. Repeat the treatment once every 3 days for as long as 3 weeks.

Another option would be a treatment that mixes 1/2 an ounce of **Almond Oil** with 400 IU's of **Vitamin E.** Warm up the mixture to body temperature and apply 1/2 an eye dropper into each affected ear. Massage the mixture within the ear and remove any excess using cotton balls. Administer this treatment for a period of six days, stop for three days, and then repeat.

Vegetable oil or olive oil are useful to clean out any debris within the ear canal. Administer using a cotton bud.

Psorinum or **Sulphur** helps relieve irritation.

Ear mites are very easy to determine. They simply look like tiny black coffee grounds within the ear canal. Your pet will shake his/her head from side to side frequently, and scratch the ears consistently if having ear mites.

Homemade Flea Spray for Dogs.

You Will Need:

- 1 cup apple cider vinegar (you can also use white distilled vinegar but the apple cider variety smells a little less harsh)
- 1 quart water
- 2-3 drops of lavender oil

Method:

Combine all ingredients in a large spray bottle. Spray along your dog's coat avoiding eyes, ears, nose and mouth. To apply to the facial area, dip a cloth in the liquid and wipe around the face. You can also spray this on their bedding to fight off fleas.

Sour Stomach: Digestive issues can be a common ailment in pets, especially older animals. If you notice your pet is making significantly more or less bathroom attempts, a simple blockage could be the problem. Try adding **canned pumpkin** or finely diced **prunes** to his/her food. Serve this for a couple of days until you notice the problem has eased. But be careful! Prune pits are toxic to animals, so make sure the prunes are pit-free.

Cracked Paws and Pads: Your dog's paws and pads can develop uncomfortable cracks for a variety of reasons such as a hot or cold pavement or foreign objects. Check the pad and remove any spurs or small pebbles that may be there. Wash gently with warm water and a cloth, and apply a gentle, fragrance free moisturizer, Magnesium oil, or petroleum jelly to the area.

Coat health: Fish oil is a simple and cost effective treatment to improve overall coat health. It will make your dog's coat shiny and soft. Apply 1-2 pumps of all natural fish oil into a kitchen spoon and let your dog lap it up, or administer with their food once daily.

Dry or Itchy Skin: Dogs can suffer from dry skin just as we do. Try applying **vitamin E** to the affected areas of the skin. You may also ease the itch with a homemade **oatmeal paste**. Add a little water to finely ground oatmeal until it forms a paste. Apply this to your dog's itchy areas, let sit for 10 minutes, then rinse thoroughly. It works wonders, and your dog will smell wonderful.

Liver Health:

Liver cancer is a common type of cancer among dogs which makes liver health management incredibly important for your canine. A healthy liver is effective at eliminating toxic waste in the body. Improve your dog's overall liver with **milk thistle.** This herb helps increase bile flow and is considered one of the best herbs for liver health. B Vitamins, unsweetened yogurt, and leafy green vegetables are also helpful with improving liver function. Look for supplements and vitamins at your specialty pet store.

Diarrhea: Loose stool can be indicative of minor stomach issues or more serious conditions. Try to remedy the symptoms of diarrhea by simply withholding food from them for 24 hours. This may tell you if something in their food is causing the issue, and if so, fasting for a day will aid to flush out toxins and other impurities from within their body. Seek help from a vet if the problem persists or seems too severe. Provide your dog with plenty of water as most of their fluids are leaving through their stool. Avoid dehydration by providing ample amounts of water or give your pet 1/2 cup of a sports drink to help balance his/her electrolytes.

Homemade Braided Dog Toy:

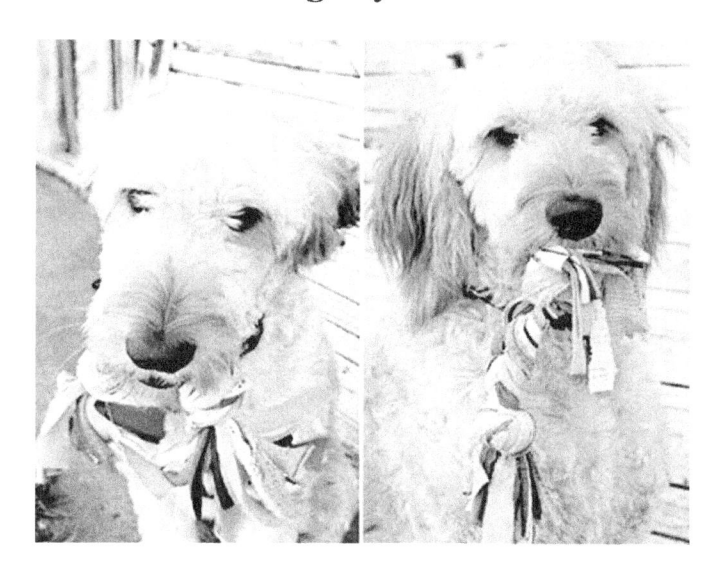

You Will Need:

- Old t-shirts
- Scissors

Make it fun by using three different shirts of various colors!

How To:

1. Cut 12-15 strips of your old t-shirt (or 4-5 strips of each t-shirt if using 3 shirts)

2. Gather all strips together and tie a tight knot at one end

3. Braid all strands together and make a knot at the bottom

Overall Nutrition:

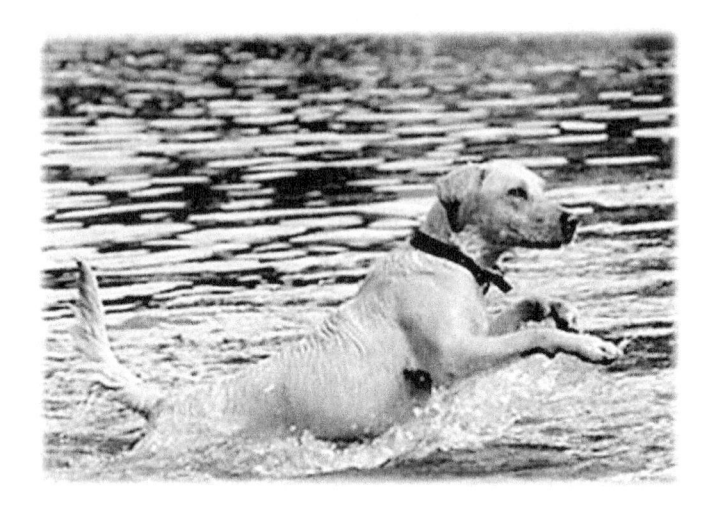

Keep your dog healthy and happy with homemade dog food and treats. Not only can you play a more active part in managing his/her weight, but you can take the guess work out of what is going into your pet's body. Proper health and weight management starts with well-balanced nutrition.

Homemade Dog Food & Treats

The recipe below is a popular choice because it is easy, makes several portions that you can store and freeze, and has over 36 grams of protein per serving!

Turkey and Vegetable Homemade Dog Food:

You will need:

- 1 cup of brown rice
- Olive oil
- 3 lbs. ground turkey
- 3 cups baby spinach
- 2 carrots (shredded)
- 1 zucchini (shredded)
- 1 cup English peas (fresh or frozen)

Method:

1. In a medium saucepan, cook rice according to the package directions and set aside.

2. Heat olive oil in large pot or Dutch oven over a medium heat. Brown the ground turkey for about 5 minutes or until cooked through.

3. Stir in the spinach, carrots, zucchini, English peas, and cooked rice. Continue to cook until heated through thoroughly which takes about 5 more minutes.

4. Let cool completely.

5. To store, separate into one cup portions, package and freeze. For meal time, just thaw in the refrigerator the night before, and microwave for 30 seconds if needed.

Canines have tastes and preferences just like we do, so try out this recipe also and see which one he likes best. It is quick, simple to make, and easy on your dog's digestive tract. Dogs are carnivores, and their digestive system works a lot differently than our own. Because of that, they can consume different types of foods such as raw meat and egg shells (for calcium). These are actually good for them! Check out this recipe below for an affordable, healthy dog food.

Chicken Casserole Homemade Dog Food:

You will need:

- 4 chicken breasts
- 1 cup green beans (roughly chopped)
- 1 cup carrots (chopped)
- 1 cup broccoli (finely chopped)
- Rolled oats
- 4 cups low sodium chicken stock

Method:

1. Start by cutting the chicken breasts into small 1 inch sized chunks.

2. Cook the chicken over a medium heat in a skillet until cooked through and no longer pink for approximately 5-7 minutes.

3. Transfer the cooked chicken to a large stock pot or Dutch oven. Add green beans, carrots, broccoli, rolled oats, and chicken broth, and cook until carrots are tender (about 15-17 minutes)

4. Let mixture cool completely before transferring to freezer safe storage containers.

Note: Keep 2-3 days' worth of food in your refrigerator thawed and ready to serve. This will help give you a head start when needing to thaw more portions. Refrigerated servings will keep for up to five days.

When making your own dog food, be sure each recipe fulfills your pup's nutrition requirements. Many homemade recipes fall short in iron, copper, calcium, and zinc, all of which are necessary for a well-balanced diet. If you think your recipe is lacking, consider adding a nutritional supplement.

If making entire meals for your dog sounds daunting, start small with homemade dog treats. Even small steps will ensure your dog's health will go a long way. Treat him/her with these wholesome, organic dog treats. The added fish oil helps improve your dog's coat health, making their coat shiny and soft.

Organic Peanut Butter Dog Treats:

You will need:

- 2 cups of organic whole wheat flour (use white flour if your dog has wheat allergies)
- 1 cup organic rolled oats
- 1 cup of water, divided

- 1/3 cup of organic creamy peanut butter (see note below to make your own)
- 1 Tablespoon honey
- Tablespoon fish oil

Method:

1. Preheat your oven to 350 degrees Fahrenheit.

2. Mix together the flour and rolled oats. Add one cup of water and blend until combined.

3. Add the peanut butter, honey, and fish oil and mix until well blended.

4. Add in the other cup of water and stir until mixture reaches a dough like consistency.

5. Lightly flour your work space, and roll the dough into a ¼ inch thick sheet. Using a pizza cutter or chef's knife, cut the dough into small cookie shapes.

6. Bake at 350 degrees for 40 minutes. Allow to cool completely before serving or storing.

7. Store in an airtight container and wait for your pup to go crazy over these!

Note: Non-organic store brands of peanut butter often contain additives, extra sweeteners and hydrogenated oils, all of which can be harmful to your pet. Opt for organic varieties or make your own! Just blend raw peanuts and peanut oil together in your food processor until smooth.

There are countless ways to bring a homemade touch to pet ownership. Don't fret about doing everything at once and start with the basics. Use these easy, simple, homemade treatments to keep your furry family member happy and healthy.

Time to cut out the junk.

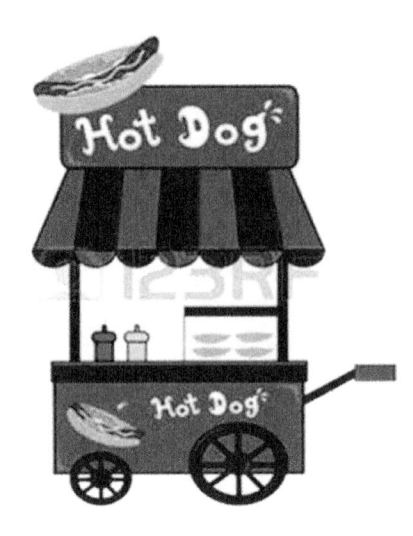

Recent statistical data has shown a rise in the number of overweight dogs throughout recent years. The good news is that there are natural remedies may help them achieve their ideal weight. In view of the concerns generated on this subject, there is a growing contention on what the 'ideal' weight for a dog should be.

You want the best for your dog and the guiding rule for each point mentioned, is to help you achieve knowledge and understanding with how to handle any weight challenges. Generally, patience is the key factor as it takes approximately 2 to 8 Months to get appreciable results on any weight loss plan you implement.

Is your dog over weight?

There are other scientific ways to know the weight of your dog, but the methods below can give you great results. Here are simple techniques you can do at home:

1. Ask your dog to lie down. This helps you get a good view from the top. The rib cage of your dog should be seen clearly followed by a waist that links the backside of your dog. If the waist is not seen, that means your dog is overweight. As long as all other parameters are in place, any dog whose waist does not show whilst lying down is overweight.

2. A side view of your dog should reveal an area that tucks in. This area is the side of the waist. However, if the tuck is not visible and the body runs parallel to the size of the chest region; then your dog is overweight. Based on these points that have been listed, you do not need to fuss about natural remedies for pets that need weight loss. A good natural and well portioned diet coupled with frequent exercise and play, is sufficient to start them on the right path.

3. The area or the base over your dog's tail must be hard. The hardness is an indication that the weight of the dog is ideal. If the base is not hard or is difficult to spot, then your dog is overweight.

4. You can hug your dog and feel its ribs. If you can easily spot the ribs with a little layer of flesh over them, then the dog has a good weight. On the other hand, if the ribs are covered with a fleshy mass; the dog is overweight. The general rule is to apply these steps once every two weeks until you get to an ideal weight that you intend to maintain for him/her.

Dog Condition Weight Chart

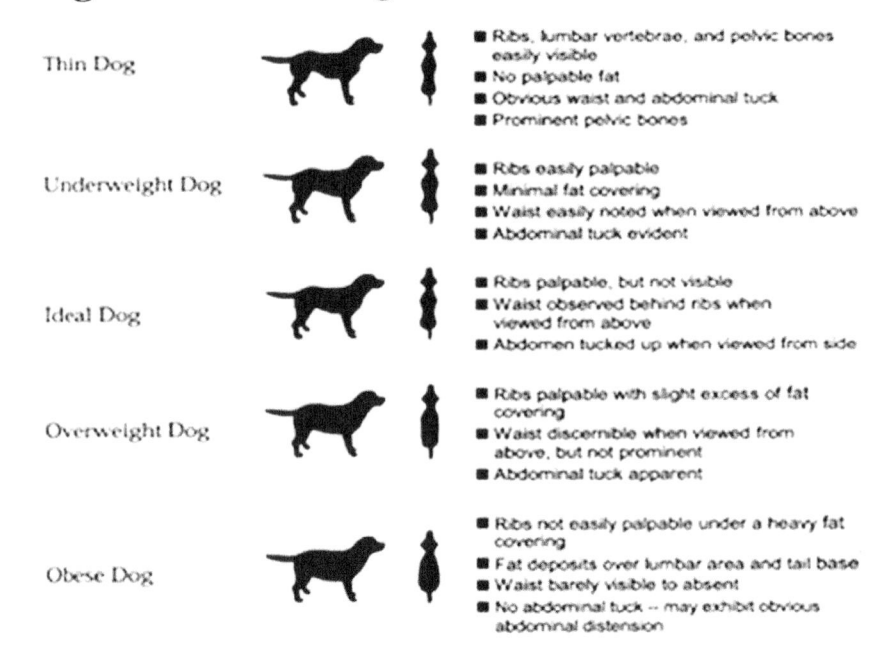

Thin Dog			■ Ribs, lumbar vertebrae, and pelvic bones easily visible ■ No palpable fat ■ Obvious waist and abdominal tuck ■ Prominent pelvic bones
Underweight Dog			■ Ribs easily palpable ■ Minimal fat covering ■ Waist easily noted when viewed from above ■ Abdominal tuck evident
Ideal Dog			■ Ribs palpable, but not visible ■ Waist observed behind ribs when viewed from above ■ Abdomen tucked up when viewed from side
Overweight Dog			■ Ribs palpable with slight excess of fat covering ■ Waist discernible when viewed from above, but not prominent ■ Abdominal tuck apparent
Obese Dog			■ Ribs not easily palpable under a heavy fat covering ■ Fat deposits over lumbar area and tail base ■ Waist barely visible to absent ■ No abdominal tuck -- may exhibit obvious abdominal distension

Factors that can lead to having an overweight Dog.

1. **Age:** Dogs do not usually have weight challenges when they are over 7 years or when they are 2 years or younger but there are very rare exceptions to this rule. The common age bracket for dog's to have weight issues stand at 2 to 6 years. This singular fact will help you understand if your dog is susceptible, or if there might be other issues affecting their health.

2. **The Breed of your Dog:** Some breeds have a stronger leaning towards being overweight than others. Dog breeds in this category include; Collies, Basset Hounds, Beagles, Cairn Terriers, Shelties, Labrador Retrievers, Cocker Spaniels and Dachshunds.

3. **A challenge in the Thyroid:** The Thyroid is the part of your dog's body that helps break down fat. If the

Thyroid is challenged, it can lead to a massive gain in weight. Medically, this is referred to as Hypothyroidism.

4. **Diet:** If your dog does not get the required nutrients he/she needs, there is the tendency for the cells in their body to react. This may leave your dog wanting to eat excessively. Your pet is simply starved of what the body naturally craves and this can lead to obesity. If you are unable to feed your dog a homemade diet, opt in for a natural balanced grain free holistic dog food.

5. **Lack of Exercise:** There are plenty of ways in which your dog burns his/her calories. The higher the goal, the more exercise they need to engage in order to obtain their ideal weight. Experts have shown the correlation between good exercise and a dog's overall lifespan. A safe rule to follow in most cases is to find out what is ideal for your pet.

Easy ways to have an effective weight loss program for your Dog.

If an overweight dog loses weight; her/she may add as much as two dog years to its lifespan. Here are a few tips:

1. **Cut back on treats between meals:** It is not healthy to give your pets snacks in between meals. Give alternative snacks such as wholesome apples, sliced carrots and boiled bones.

2. **A good exercise routine:** There are so many games that you can play with your pet to help him/her burn calories and increase their metabolism. A brisk walk, jogging, playing fetch, or taking them to the dog park.

The good thing about exercise is that it allows you to bond while adding health benefits to your pet.

3. **Weight Management:** Feeding your dog twice daily with the right calorie intake, will helps them to achieve their ideal weight.

Get it right from the onset: The ideal weight loss plan will help your dog lose approximately 1 to 2% of its body fat per week. Some pet owners put into action routines that offer a higher weight loss result per week but this can be detrimental to your pet. Your pet may lose muscle and essential tissue if you push them too hard, so doing this, may result in health complications.

Processed foods: There are some pet foods that claim to give your dog the edge they need for a good weight loss plan. However, careful research shows that the components used in making some of these products could do more harm than good. If you really want the best for your dog, it's best to stick to a disciplined meal and exercise program that works slowly over time.

A Healthy Weight Loss Product Combination: Your dog's food must have a below average calorie intake, above the average protein, and below the average fat. Protein makes your pet feel full and gives him/her the right nutrients it needs.

What to do if you have more than one dog: It is important to create a plan to feed your overweight dog in a separate space. Monitor what he/she eats and keep track of the progress being made.

Healthy recipes for your Dog.

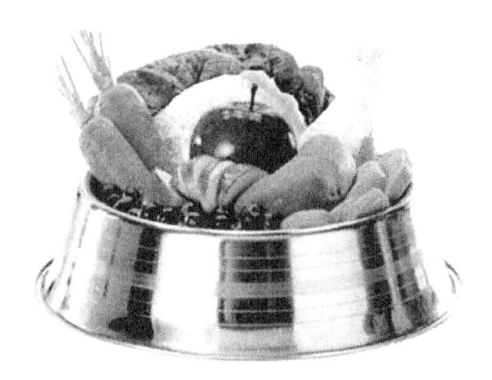

Rice, Chicken and Broccoli Meal.

This recipe is ideal for your dog as a balanced meal, broccoli can be served as a snack or incorporated into part of their meal. It is rich in calcium and helps to promote fresh breath.

What you need:

- 5 Pounds of diced chicken.
- 1 whole chicken can be used for this recipe and this includes the liver, the neck meat and the heart.
- Skinless/boneless chicken Breasts can also spice things up if this is your preference.
- 5 Whole eggs (These can be cooked or raw)
- 5 Cups of Rice (whole grain as this is highly nutritional
- Chopped broccoli (approximately 3 Cups)
- 3 Tbsp. of olive oil

Method:

1. Boil the rice and chicken for approximately 30-40 minutes. Ensure that the chicken is almost fully cooked before you introduce the broccoli. Simmer the broccoli for 2 to 3 Minutes. Add the broccoli to the chicken and rice when the chicken is ready to be served. Allow the meal to cool down before adding the olive oil and eggs.

2. You can store the remainder of the food in the fridge using an airtight container for up to for 5 days.

Tips: Olive Oil does not contain high cholesterol which makes it good for the heart and overall health of your dog. Whole grains help to keep their cells active which in turn, aids in breaking down excess fat.

Dried Chicken Jerk Recipe.

You can give your pet a treat with this meal. It is easy to prepare, and is packed with nutrition.

What you need:

- 2 chicken breast is sufficient for an average serving.

Method:

1. The oven needs to be preheated to 200 degrees Fahrenheit.

2. The chicken breasts should be sliced into 1/8 inch thick strips with the use of a paring knife. The chicken breasts should be turned on their side and all excess fat from the chicken must be drained.

3. Carefully place the strips on a baking sheet and bake for 2 hours.

4. The chicken must be dry before it is removed from the oven. It must not be soft and chewy. When it is completely cool, it can be served to your pet.

5. The jerky can be stored for a maximum of 2 weeks in an airtight container.

Chicken and Vegetable Dinner:

This recipe comes with a rich source of minerals and vitamins from the vegetables, and the chicken provides plenty of protein. It also helps dogs that need to lose a few pounds since the fatty part of the chicken can easily be removed.

What you need:

- 4 Cups of Water
- Chopped Carrots (1 Cup)
- Chopped Green Beans (1 Cup)
- 1 Tablespoon of Fish Oil (Optional)
- 2 Cups of Brown Rice
- 1 Pound of Ground Chicken

Method:

1. The ground chicken should be cooked in a non-stick skillet on medium heat. This should take about 30 to 35 minutes to cook thoroughly.

2. Add the chicken, brown rice, and water in a large Pot. Boil until the rice is cooked.

3. Reduced to simmer until the rice is ready to serve. This takes approximately 15 minutes.

4. Add the green beans and carrots and cook for 2 minutes until it is soft and tender.

5. Allow to cool, then serve.

6. It can be stored in the fridge within an airtight container for up to 5 days.

Tips: Don't use heavy oil on the chicken. You can use canola, olive oil, or other low cholesterol oils.

Chicken Casserole:

The vegetables in this recipe help to give your dog a healthy intestinal tract, the green beans help make them feel full. The protein and other vitamins makes for a healthy recipe.

What you need:

- 4 Cups of Low-Salt Chicken Broth
- 4 Chicken Breasts
- Half Cup of Chopped Carrot
- Half Cup of Chopped Broccoli
- Half Cup of Rolled Oats
- Half Cup of Chopped Green Beans

Method:

1. Remove all excess fat from the chicken breasts. Cut the chicken into small chunks.

2. Cook the chicken in a non-stick skillet on medium heat until it is no longer pink. This takes about 25 to 30 Minutes.

3. Add the chicken broth, vegetables, chicken, and rolled oats into a large pot and cook on medium heat for approximately 15 minutes until the carrots become tender.

4. Allow to cool before serving.

5. You can store this in the fridge using an airtight container for up to 5 days.

6. A little amount of olive oil can be used to fry the chicken breasts.

Grocery Shopping List for Dogs.

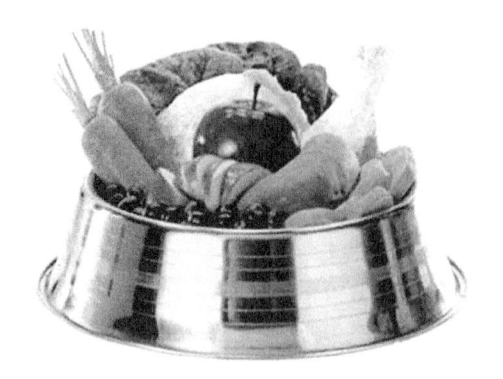

Meat.

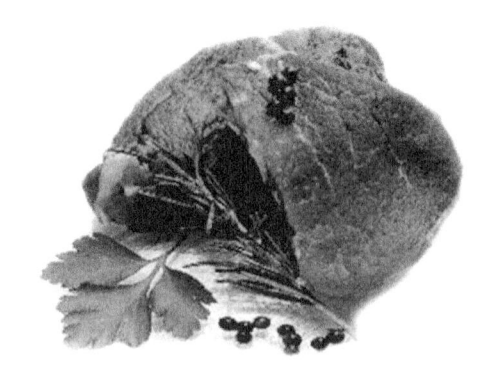

Ground Turkey
Whole Chicken/Breasts

Produce.

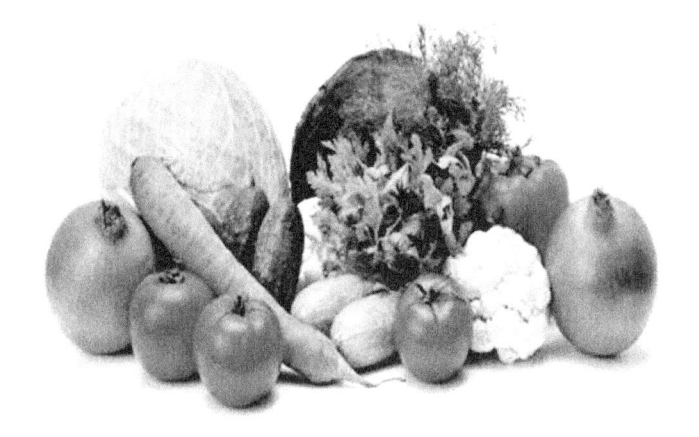

Spinach (baby)
Green Beans
Broccoli
Zucchini
Peas (English)
Fruit (your choice)
Carrots
Parsley
Mint

Poultry.

Eggs

Grains/Nuts/Other.

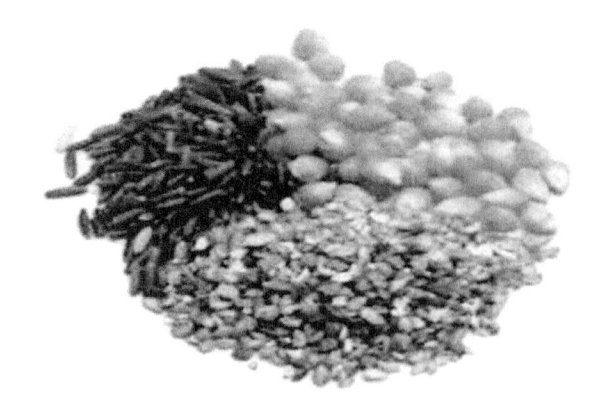

Brown Rice
Oats
Wheat Flour
Brown Rice Flour
Peanut Butter
Honey
Fish Oil
Olive Oil
Charcoal
Chlorophyll (liquid)

Dogs with Asthma: What you need to know

Asthma is simply your pet's reaction to certain allergens. Some of these allergic reactions may be caused by air pollutants such as dust or pollen. Symptoms may also occur through certain types of ingredients in their diet. The initial symptoms may begin with wheezing and coughing. Most dogs that suffer from allergies are usually in adulthood through a weakness in their immune system, or a breakdown in their body's defense mechanism. There are other factors that can lead to asthma such as cancer, or infections with worms and other viral foreign bodies. Some dog breeds such as the Maltese and Pug, are prone to asthma due to restricted construction of their airway passages.

Tips on how to manage it:

Invest in air purifiers and place them in each room of your home. Close windows during the spring season when pollen is at its worst. Even simple activities such as cutting your grass (if windows are open) may bring about an asthma attack for your pet. Although fresh homemade food is always the healthiest diet, if you buy processed food, your pet may be allergic to certain ingredients within it such as grains. Allergy free, holistic food is the best way to go.

Keep your house clean by regularly dusting and vacuuming to keep pollutants at a minimum.

Herbal Remedies.

The Wonders of Natural Black Seed Oil:

Natural Black seed Oil has many ingredients that have made it a product of choice for many pet owners. It is a plant in which oil is extracted and produced in capsule format. There are many health benefits that black seed oil can benefit from which include; allergies, an overactive immune system, asthma, intestinal disorders, coughs, and cold and flu symptoms. Black Seed oil holds anti-inflammatory properties and can be used as a preventive measure for your pet.

How to administer:

1 tsp. can be given to your pet once per day for 3 days and then reduced to one tsp. every 2 week when the immune system has fully bounced back. Some pets have a negative reaction to black seed oil so keep a watchful eye out and discontinue use if vomiting occurs, or if you notice any other abnormal reactions.

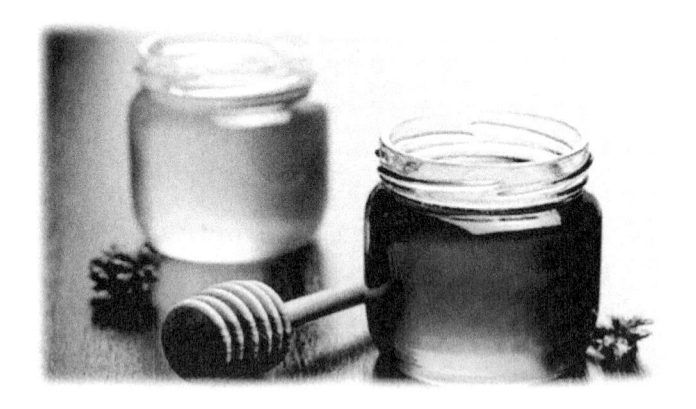

CHAMOMILE TEA.

Eye Ailments

This traditional medicinal tea has made history for thousands of years for its natural ability to calm mental conditions such as anxiety and unsettling stomach ailments. Chamomile also has the natural ability to help soothe aching and dry eyes.

Method:

- Put one chamomile tea bag in a glass of hot water. Let it steep for 5 minutes.
- Take out the tea bag and then place it in a glass of cold water for another 5 minutes.
- Take it out and dry the remaining liquid a little.
- Gently hold the tea bag on to your dog's eyes for 3 to 5 minutes.

OATMEAL.

Irritated/itchy Skin

- Oatmeal has the natural ability to cure skin ailments. It can also be used to treat irritated, dry, and itchy skin.

Method:

1. Mix oatmeal (fine grind) with a little water until it becomes a paste.
2. Apply it on the irritated areas and leave for 10 minutes.
3. Rinse with warm water.

CANNED PUMPKIN.

Better Digestion for Constipation

Pumpkin is rich in fiber, low in fat, and cholesterol, it is also loaded with beta carotene, magnesium, potassium, iron, zinc, and vitamins A and C. It has the benefit of soothing the digestive tract. Whether it is a metabolic disorder, or neuromuscular diseases that lead to constipation, organic canned pumpkin can help. This diet contains high fiber that assists in a better colon movement to ease symptoms.

Method:

Buy organic canned pumpkin from your nearest grocery store.

Serve half a can in the morning, and half the can at night until symptoms subside.

DANDELION.

Digestive System

Dandelion is French in origin, a word meaning 'lion's tooth'. Dandelion is rich in vitamin A, C, iron, and calcium. It provides soft stimulation to the digestive system and aids in the removal of waste. It is beneficial for both colon cleansing as well as the urinary tract. Dandelion is highly diuretic in nature therefore aiding with gallbladder and kidney detoxification. Due to its rich calcium content, dandelion has the ability to protect bones and help slow down the aging process.

Method:

1. One spoon of dandelion tea powder mixed into a 6 oz. cup of hot water.

2. Stir well and let it steep for approximately 5 minutes.

3. Wait for the temperature to drop before serving it to your dog.

ALOE VERA.

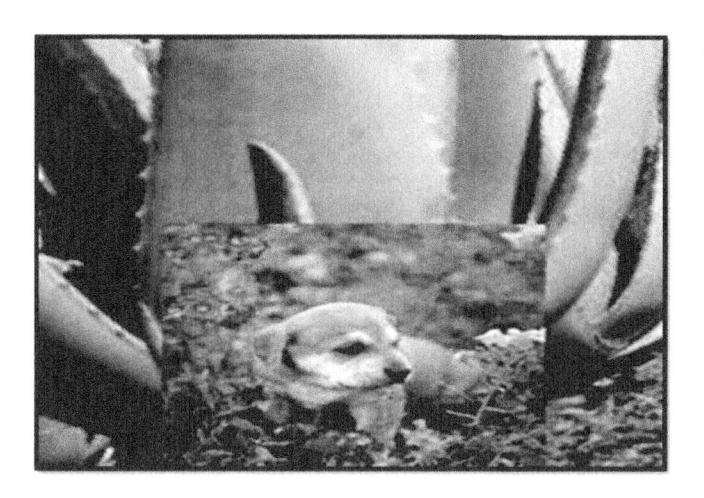

Inflammation and Abrasions

This natural herbal plant has history dating back 6,000 years. Aloe Vera has been traditionally used as a remedy for its soothing and healing properties on burns and scrapes and is safe use for pets. It is used to treat skin wounds and reduce inflammation.

Method:

1. Cut the Aloe Vera leaf in half.

2. Use a knife to score the inside of the leave to release the gel and apply.

HONEY.

If you find it hard to find natural aloe Vera, you can always opt in for honey as a replacement to treat burns and scrapes. Honey is also a natural energy booster. Its non-preservative sugar has the ability to prevent fatigue during exercise. While Manuka honey from New Zealand is the best choice, other kinds of natural honey can do just as well. Honey contains anti-oxidant and antibacterial properties that helps treat several skin conditions.

Method:

Apply to the area and leave on for 20 minutes before rinsing.

GREEN TEA.

Boosting the Immune System

The incredible benefits of green tea has been well documented. Its contains a substance that works on a cellular level to protect cells and molecules from damage. It can benefit your dog by stimulating and boosting his/her immune system. It also acts as an anti-oxidant agent as well as an astringent to help cure stomach and skin cancer. The antioxidant Epigallocatechin Gallate (EGCG) is one of the most powerful compounds contained in this natural remedy.

CORN SILK

Blood Pressure and Bladder ailments

Corn Silk was believed to have been cultivated by the Aztecs and Mayans. It bears a diuretic natural ability to help animals with bladder or urinary tract infection. It contains proteins, fiber, as well as an ample supply of vitamins to aid the treatment of waste removal complications. It can also help lower your dog's blood pressure.

CARROTS

Colon Disorders

Carrots are high in fiber and rich with vitamin C and can be used as a natural herbal treatment for your pet. Finely blended, or grated carrots mixed in with your dog's food will help illuminate mucus that houses parasites inside the colon. Carrots are extremely beneficial to help fight infection within the body.

LICORICE ROOT

Liver Detoxification

This particular herb aids in the detoxification of the liver tissue and also helps fight liver disease. It helps to cure ulcers in the digestive system by promoting cell regrowth. Dogs with eczema can also benefit from Licorice Root. However, be advised that licorice is not suitable if your dog is pregnant or has a heart condition.

Method:

Finely chop the dried licorice root and place inside an empty jar.

Pour olive oil on top of the licorice root until you can see the liquid layer is ½" above the herb.

Close the jar tight and place it away from sunlight for a month.

After a month, strain the oil through a sieve and apply.

ALFALFA

Arthritis, Cancer and Bladder Irritation

Alfalfa contains a variety of minerals including; iron, calcium, magnesium, copper, potassium, folate, phosphorous, zinc and silicon. It is also rich with protein and contains vitamins A, B, C, D, E and K. Alfalfa also helps with arthritis, cancer and bladder irritation.

Method:

1. Use powdered alfalfa's leaves or sprouted seeds.
2. Mix 1 teaspoon into your dog's food twice daily.

BURDOOK ROOT

Blood Cleanser

This native herb is derived from Northern Europe and Siberia and is considered by many vets as extremely effective. The root is low in calories and contains small amounts of electrolyte potassium. If you live in an area where it is difficult to find this plant, opt in for dried root or tincture. It acts as both an antioxidant and blood cleanser.

Method:

1. Add 1 teaspoon of burdock root and 1 cup of water to a pot and boil it.
2. Reduce the heat and simmer for another 15 minutes.
3. Strain it through a sieve and place it into in an air tight container.

4. Mix 1 tablespoon with your dog's food per day, and serve.

CALENDULA Oil

Helps treat inflammation of wounds

This wonderful plant extract has natural healing abilities and also acts as a pain reliever. Its properties acts as an astringent, has antibacterial agents, it is antifungal, antiviral, and antimicrobial. It is generally used to treat wounds, abrasions and mouth inflammation. Whilst helping with tissue regrowth, calendula oil also tones down swelling in the mouth and throat. It can also help treat pain of ear infections. Some studies suggest that Calendula has a faster recovery rate than that of Aloe Vera gel.

Method:

1. Place the dried calendula blossoms and olive oil into a jar.
2. Tightly close the jar and leave in sunlight for 2 weeks.
3. Strain and store the oil in the dark place.
4. Use the oil accordingly.

GINGER

Intestinal Gas

The benefits of Ginger serves as an enhancer in blood circulation and sweating. It provides stimulation to various organs. Ginger consists of the essential oils; beta-carotene, acetic acid, alpha-linolenic acid, ascorbic acid, camphor, capsaicin, and gingerol. Ginger also acts as a soothing agent within the intestinal tract eliminating intestinal gas.

Method:

1. Peel the skin and finely chop the Ginger.
2. Mix 1/2 tsp. for small dog, and 1 tsp. for medium/large breeds.

LEMON BALM LEAVES

Fresh Breath and also Anxiety

Lemon Balm is a member of the mint family, it helps with bad breath problem. The color of this herb ranges from dark green to a yellowish green. It contains the ingredients; volatile oils, tannins, and flavonoids. It can address several issues in your dog such as; stress, anxiety, sleep disorder and depression.

Method:

1. Place 2 tablespoons of freshly chopped lemon balm leaves into a cup of warm water.
2. Stir for a while and serve.

MULLEIN

Insect Bites and Minor Wounds

Mullein is useful for treating insect bites and minor wounds. This natural herb consists of mucilage and small amounts of Saponins and Tannins

Method:

1. Chop the mullein leaves finely then mix with a spoonful of water.

2. Gently apply to the affected area.

NEIM

Insect Repellent/Skin Irritation

This natural herbal extract can relieve sunburn, itchy paws, and act as an insect repellent. It also has anti-inflammatory qualities that can help soothe skin irritations.

Method:

1. Add 1 1/2 teaspoons of dried Neim leaves into a cup of warm water.

2. Let it sit overnight.

3. Strain the tea over a sieve then pour the tea into an empty spray bottle.

4. Spray on to the affected area as needed.

NETTLE

Helps Blood Clotting and also acts as an Antibacterial Agent

Nettle has antibacterial, astringent and antihistamine properties. It plays an important role in most dog's skin conditions. It can also help with nosebleeds, or other hemorrhagic conditions.

Method:

1. For blood clotting, add 1/2 a teaspoon of dried grinded nettle into your dog's food.

2. To aid in irritated skin conditions, try using nettle as a rinse.

3. Mix 1 tablespoon of dried nettle with 1 cup of boiling water.

4. Let it sit for 5 minutes and then strain the liquid. Use the liquid as a rinse after shampoo.

PARSLEY

Arthritis/lower Blood Pressure

Parsley is rich in fiber, protein, and vitamins, and has great healing properties for dogs. It consists of volatile oil such as Myristicin, Limonene, Eugenol, and Alpha-thujene. It also contains flavonoids that includes Apiin, Apigenin, Crisoeriol, and Luteolin which are agents that aid inflammation as well as help fight arthritis and cancer. Since it is also diuretic, it can also help fight urinary tract disorders and lower blood pressure.

Method:

1. Boil 4 glasses of water.

2. Add 1 small bowl of fresh parsley into the boiling water.

3. Cover and turn off the stove and let it sit for 3 to 4 hours.

4. Turn the stove back on and simmer on low heat for 1 hour.

5. Open the cover and release the heat and strain the leaves.

6. Cool down in the refrigerator before serving to your dog.

ROSE TEA

Skin and Digestive ailments

Method:

1. Use the petals only and place in a cup then pour the hot water to drown the petals.

2. Let sit for 20 minutes then strain the petals.

3. 1 tablespoon of rose tea twice daily can aid in your dog's upset stomach.

4. You may also use rose tea to clean cuts or abrasions.

Index

A

Acidophilus	68
allergies	1, 30, 32, 33, 35, 50, 52, 76, 85, 101, 102
ALOE VERA	105
Amaranth	26
amino acids	21, 26, 35, 47
Apple Cider Vinegar	34, 56
Ascorbate Acid	48

B

bad breath	43, 72, 110
BEER YEAST	11
Bilberry	7
Black Seed Oil	102
Black walnut	69
bladder	44, 45, 46, 56, 106, 108
BLUEBERRY	8

C

Calendula	32, 33, 109
Cayenne pepper	68
CHAMOMILE	103
Chicory Root	26
Chlorophyll	72, 73, 100
Chromium	7, 8
CHROMIUM PICOLINATE	8
cloves	12
coconut oil	50, 53, 70, 71
Colloidal Silver	48
cranberry	44, 56

D

DANDELION	104
depression	6, 110
diabetes	1, 4, 5, 6, 7, 8, 9, 10, 11, 17, 18
Diabetic recipes	11
diarrhea	29, 30, 37, 57, 77, 80
Diatomaceous	67

E

Ear Mites	77
Echinacea	47
Exercise	18, 58, 91

F

Fennel	67
FENUGREEK SEEDS	9
Fiber	8, 28
fruit	8, 23, 24, 68

K

Kidney Health	56

L

lavender oil	50, 78
lemon Eucalyptus	56
Licorice Root	33, 107
Linoleic Acid	26
Liver Health	80
Lubricants	28
Lyceum	47

M

minerals 11, 26, 35, 95, 108
Mouth Wash 71

N

NOPAL CACTUS 9

O

OMEGA 3 9
Oregon grape holly 46

P

Parsley 43, 63, 67, 69, 73, 99, 112
PLANTAGO OVATA 7
Probiotics 68
Propolis 43, 48
protein 7, 13, 21, 24, 37, 59, 83, 92, 95, 96, 108, 112
Psorinum 78
Pumpkin seeds 66

R

Rosemary 25, 63

S

Sage 26, 43, 63
Shopping List for Cats 62
Shopping List for Dogs 98
Soy Lecithin 25

T

Thyme	26
Thyroid	90
ticks	52, 56
Toothpaste	43
TURMERIC ROOT	10

V

Vitamin C	46, 48

W

Weight Chart	90
Weight loss	5
Wheat germ oil	66
Wormwood oil	67

Y

yellow dock	77

Author

Pennie Mae Cartawick is an author of both fiction and nonfiction books. Her work is based on a variety of subjects including weight management and nutrition, recipe books, horror novelettes, and short Sherlock Holmes mysteries to name a few. She also draws her own illustrations for some of her short stories such as in "Silence Be Damned" and "The EXCHANGE". Her nonfiction books "Choosing the Right Diet for Success" and "The DETOX CLOCK" achieved the top 100 best seller list within the first week of publication.

She was born in the city of Sheffield in South Yorkshire England. Shortly after graduating high school, she worked as a Model and attended Shirecliffe College for Drama. Thereafter, she attended Stannington College for English, Art, communication skills and Photography. She then moved to London in her early 20's, where she studied and attained a career as a Beauty Therapist. She also obtained various certifications at DaneGlow International for slimming wraps and other deep heat treatments, and Thalgo Cosmetics for Makeup (a French Company focusing on Marine cosmetics). Her specialized skills include Makeup, Swedish massage, Reflexology, Nutrition, diet and exercise.

She Migrated to Florida in 1993 where she has been living ever since. Although her profession Now-a-days is as a Real Estate Investor and a free-lance beauty consultant, her passion is writing, and uses the knowledge she acquired throughout the years on various subjects to enlighten others.

She is the youngest sibling of three, Anthony and Mark Cartawick.

Books

Choosing the Right Diet for Success

The DETOX CLOCK

7 Day Detox Smoothie Diet

THE FAST DIET

Detox for the Soul

SILENCE BE DAMNED

The EXCHANGE

Ghost Stories

SHERLOCK HOLMES: The Mystery of the Faceless Bride

SHERLOCK HOLMES: The Mystery of the Poisoned Tomb

SHERLOCK HOLMES: A Strange Affair with the Woman on the Tracks

SHERLOCK HOLMES: The Case of the Cracked Mirror

SHERLOCK HOLMES: The Game of Cat and Mouse

SHERLOCK HOLMES: The Curse of a Native

SHERLOCK HOLMES: The Case of the missing Mayan Codices

SHERLOCK HOLMES: Murders on the Voyage to India

SHERLOCK HOLMES: The Sphinx Collection

SHERLOCK HOLMES: The Phoenix Collection

SHERLOCK HOLMES: The Ultimate Satyr Collection

SHERLOCK HOLMES: The Heist

SHERLOCK HOLMES: Death in the Tropics of an English Explorer

SHERLOCK HOLMES: Dirty Laundry in Paradise

SHERLOCK HOLMES: Watson to the Rescue

SHERLOCK HOLMES: NOT SO MERRY IN GOOD OL' SCOTLAND

SHERLOCK HOLMES: Mysterious Murders Surround the Whistling Tavern

Printed in Great Britain
by Amazon